BSAVA
Pocketbook
for Vets

second edition

Editor:
Sheldon Middleton
MA VetMB MRCVS

T0203153

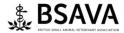

BSAVA
BRITISH SMALL ANIMAL VETERINARY ASSOCIATION

Published by:
British Small Animal Veterinary Association
Woodrow House, 1 Telford Way, Waterwells Business Park,
Quedgeley, Gloucester GL2 2AB

A Company Limited by Guarantee in England.
Registered Company No. 2837793.
Registered as a Charity.

First printed 2019
Reprinted 2020, 2021 twice, 2022

A catalogue record for this book is available from the British Library.

ISBN 978-1-910443-61-3

The publishers, editors and contributors cannot take responsibility for
information provided on dosages and methods of application of drugs
mentioned or referred to in this publication. Details of this kind must
be verified in each case by individual users from up to date literature
published by the manufacturers or suppliers of those drugs. Veterinary
surgeons are reminded that in each case they must follow all
appropriate national legislation and regulations (for example, in the
United Kingdom, the prescribing cascade) from time to time in force.

Printed by Zenith Media, Pontypool NP4 0DQ.
Printed on ECF paper made from sustainable forests.

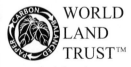

WORLD
LAND
TRUST™

www.carbonbalancedpaper.com
CBP013789

Carbon Balancing is delivered by World Land Trust, an international
conservation charity, who protects the world's most biologically
important and threatened habitats acre by acre. Their Carbon
Balanced Programme offsets emissions through the purchase and
preservation of high conservation value forests.

17595PUBS22

Other BSAVA Member benefits

For further information on any of the below benefits of membership email administration@bsava.com, or call 01452 726700.

- **Congress discount**
  All members enjoy substantial discounts on Congress registration which is automatically applied when you book online.

- **Publications discount**
  Members save £30 on BSAVA veterinary manuals and £20 on veterinary nursing manuals.

- **Congress podcasts**
  The Congress podcast archive contains all podcasts from Congress 2011 onwards. Video and audio podcasts are available featuring our most recent content.

- **CPD discount**
  High standards and low costs are the BSAVA's key aims when delivering CPD throughout the UK. We send the annual brochure to members in advance of the general release so you won't miss out on the course you want.

- ***BSAVA Small Animal Formulary***
  This indispensable pocket guide is now in its 9th edition. Every vet member receives a free copy when they join and a free copy of each new edition. Also available online and as a smartphone app for vet members (login required for both).

- ***BSAVA Guide to Procedures in Small Animal Practice***
  This guide provides practical, step-by-step guidance on how to perform the diagnostic and therapeutic procedures commonly carried out in small animal veterinary practice.

- ***Journal of Small Animal Practice***
  Members enjoy free subscription to the digital edition of the Journal of Small Animal Practice (JSAP) which provides all the latest research and scientific advancements within the profession.

- **Companion**
  This essential monthly publication for all BSAVA members provides practical content which relates to your needs in practice. Companion delivers accessible, instructive CPD features, articles on the issues that are facing the profession and of course, general Association news.

■ **Access to the PDP Resource Bank**
Providing a range of online webinars, podcasts and articles, matched directly to each of the RCVS PDP competences.

■ **Client Information Leaflets**
Give your clients the best advice by downloading BSAVA client information leaflets. Leaflets are arranged into categories for Medicines, Behaviours, Exotic Pets and PetSavers guides.

■ **Regional CPD meetings**
BSAVA has 12 regions covering the UK, run by committed volunteers. Members can access regional CPD at reduced prices, meet other local professionals and even get involved in choosing the subjects covered in the programme.

■ **Professional representation**
At a time when the profession is subject to so much change and scrutiny, it has never been more important to make sure your views are represented at the highest level. Every time the Association takes part in a consultation, our members' views are canvassed and considered in the BSAVA's response.

■ **BSAVA Library**
The BSAVA Library contains all the Association's digital content including all the manuals, the Small Animal Formulary, Companion magazine, Congress Proceedings, client resources, scientific resources and themed collections of content.

■ **Loyalty reward gift**
Members will qualify for a loyalty reward gift each year that they renew their paid membership.

Contents

- **Foreword** ix
- **Preface** x
- **A few notes on using this book** xi

■ **A**
- Abdomen – abdominocentesis 1
- Abdominal swelling – diagnostic work-up 4
- Acepromazine 6
- Acid–base disturbances – interpreting results 7
- Acid–base disturbances – metabolic causes 7
- Acid–base disturbances – respiratory causes 8
- Adrenaline 8
- Amitriptyline 9
- Amlodipine 10
- Amoxicillin 11
- Ampicillin 13
- Anaphylaxis – emergency treatment 14
- Anorexia in rabbits – an approach to evaluation 16
- Anticoagulant rodenticide poisoning 18
- Apomorphine 21
- Arterial thrombo-embolism key points 22
- ASA physical status and classifications scale 23
- Aspirin 24
- Atipamezole 24
- Azotaemia differentiation 26

■ **B**
- Benazepril 28
- Blood glucose in rabbits 30
- Body condition scoring scheme – cats 32
- Body condition scoring scheme – dogs 34
- Bodyweight to body surface area conversion 36
- Bromhexine 38
- Buprenorphine 39
- Butorphanol 40

■ **C**
- Cabergoline 43
- Carbimazole 43
- Cardiopulmonary resuscitation 44
- Cardiopulmonary resuscitation – drugs 46
- Cardiovascular emergency sedation protocols 47
- Carprofen 48
- Cefalexin 50
- Cefovecin 51
- Charcoal 52
- Chinchilla biological data 53
- Chlorphenamine 54
- Chocolate/caffeine poisoning 54
- Cimetidine 56
- Clindamycin 58
- Co-amoxiclav 59
- Codeine 61
- Collapse 62
- Congestive heart failure – acute stabilization 63
- Corneal ulcers – causes 63
- Cranial draw test 64
- Cranial nerve tests 66
- Cystocentesis 67

■ D
— Decontamination   69
— Delmadinone   73
— Dental recording chart
  – cat   74
— Dental recording chart
  – dog   75
— Dexamethasone   76
— Dexmedetomidine   78
— Diazepam   80
— Doxycycline   82
— Drug distribution
  categories   83
— Dystocia – general
  approach   86
— Dystocia in queens   88

■ E
— Ear disease – topical
  polypharmaceuticals   90
— ECG standard leads, lead II
  diagram and reference
  ranges   91
— Endotracheal tube sizes   93
— Enrofloxacin   93
— Ethylene glycol poisoning   95

■ F
— FAST scan – abdominal   99
— Fenbendazole   101
— Ferret biological data   105
— Fipronil   105
— Firocoxib   107
— Fluids – composition of
  intravenous fluids   108
— Fluids – estimating
  percentage of
  dehydration   109
— Fluralaner   109
— Fly strike in the rabbit   110
— Furosemide   111

■ G
— Gabapentin   114
— Gastric dilatation–
  volvulus radiographic
  appearance   114
— Gerbil biological data   115
— Gestation periods in the
  bitch and queen   116
— Glaucoma – common
  causes   116
— Grape/raisin/sultana
  poisoning   117
— Guinea pig biological
  data   119

■ H
— Hamster biological data   121
— Head trauma – an approach
  to management   123
— Heart murmur grading   124
— Heart radiograph – 'clock
  face' analogy   125
— Heart rate – reference
  values   126
— Heart – vertebral heart
  score   127
— Hyperadrenocorticism   128
— Hypertension   130
— Hypoglycaemia   132

■ I
— Imidacloprid   135
— Insulin   136
— Intraocular pressure
  normal values   139
— IRIS staging – acute
  kidney injury   139
— IRIS staging – chronic
  kidney disease   140
— Ivermectin   141

■ K
- Ketamine   144
- Ketamine CRI for a 2 kg rabbit undergoing surgery   146

■ L
- Lactulose   148
- Levothyroxine   148
- Lidocaine   150
- Lipid infusions   151
- Lufenuron   152

■ M
- Maropitant   154
- Medetomidine   155
- Meloxicam   156
- Metaflumizone   158
- Methadone   158
- Methimazole   159
- Methoprene   159
- Metoclopramide   160
- Metronidazole   161
- Milbemycin   163
- Modified Glasgow coma scale   164
- Mouse biological data   165
- Moxidectin   166

■ N
- Neck pain – clinical approach   168
- Neurological examination   170
- NSAID poisoning   174

■ O
- Oclacitinib   177
- Oesophagostomy tube placement   178
- Omeprazole   182
- Ortolani test   182
- Otitis externa/media – clinical approach   185
- Oxytetracycline   186
- Oxytocin   187

■ P
- Pain scoring – cat   190
- Pain scoring – dog   192
- Paracetamol   194
- Paracetamol poisoning   195
- Patellar luxations – grading   197
- Percentage solutions conversion table   197
- Pericardial effusion key points   198
- Pimobendan   199
- Polyuria and polydipsia – diagnostic approach   200
- Potassium salts   202
- Praziquantel   203
- Pre-anaesthetic drug combinations   206
- Prednisolone   210
- Prescribing cascade   212
- Prescription – standard form   215
- Pruritus – cat   216
- Pruritus – dog   217
- Pruritus scale   218
- Pyoderma – investigation of clinical signs   220
- Pyrantel   222

■ **R**
– Rabbit biological data   225
– Rabbit reproduction
  – common owner
  concerns   226
– Ranitidine   228
– Rat biological data   228
– Respiratory distress   230
– Resting energy
  requirement   232
– Robenacoxib   232

■ **S**
– Schirmer tear test   235
– Sedation combinations   236
– Sedation of fractious cats
  and dogs   242
– Selamectin   244
– Shock – classification
  scheme   244
– Shock – general approach
  to diagnostic testing   245
– Skin lesions   246
– Spinal trauma   247
– Spinosad   248
– Status epilepticus   249
– Sucralfate   253
– Suture patterns   254
– Suture sizes   257

■ **T**
– Telmisartan   259
– Thoracocentesis   260
– Tibial compression test   262
– Tracheostomy   263
– Tramadol   265
– Tremors – differential
  diagnoses   266
– Trilostane   266

■ **U**
– Urethral catheterization
  – male cat   268
– Urinalysis – dog and
  cat   270
– Urinalysis – rabbit   271
– Urine specific gravity   272
– Uveitis causes   273

■ **W**
– Wounds – emergency
  care   277
– Wounds – recognition
  and treatment   278

■ **X**
– Xylitol poisoning   281

■ **References**   **285**
■ **Index of trade names**   **287**
■ **Emergency doses**   **292**

Foreword

BSAVA Manuals provide a wealth of practical and detailed knowledge on a wide variety of companion animal subjects, including medicine, surgery, behaviour and practice management. They are invaluable when you need to read up on a particular procedure, disease or technique in detail. However, there are times when you just need a few facts and figures, or a quick reminder of a procedure that you do infrequently or in a less familiar species.

Einstein famously said "Never memorize something that you can look up" and the *BSAVA Pocketbook for Vets* is a great aid memoire for algorithms, tests, dosages and biological data essential in day to day first opinion practice. It is a perfect size to carry around in your scrub top pocket or occupy a prominent position on your consulting room desk.

This new and updated edition is an ideal companion to the *BSAVA Small Animal Formulary*, the *BSAVA Guides to Procedures in Small Animal Practice*, *Radiographic Positioning* and *Canine and Feline Common Poisons* and the *BSAVA Pocketbook for Veterinary Nurses* – all of which are designed to be extremely practical and used on a daily basis. This is a 'must have' for new graduates and old fogeys alike, and the editor should be congratulated on producing such a useful and comprehensive book.

Philip Lhermette
BSc(Hons) CBiol FRSB BVetMed FRCVS
BSAVA President (2018–2019)

Preface

This is the second edition of the *BSAVA Pocketbook for Vets* and builds on the success of the first edition. Feedback was received that more quick reference emergency information would be useful in the book and as such more of this type of information has been included, where available. There has been a significant advance in both the science of veterinary medicine and the materials available from BSAVA in the 6 years between editions. Hopefully this book catches the essence of these advances and presents them to the reader in a user-friendly way.

Once again, I would like to thank the publications department of BSAVA for their help in producing this book and the authors whose work I have referenced.

Hopefully the format remains practical and accessible enough that it allows quick access to essential information. I have made good use of the notes section in my own copy, which has informed this edition and I would encourage others to adapt their own versions to suit their particular area of practice.

All feedback is welcome at **publications@bsava.com**.

Sheldon Middleton
MA VetMB MRCVS

Bedford
October 2018

Sheldon graduated from the University of Cambridge in 2007. He stayed in the area as a new graduate, taking a job in a mixed practice in Bedford. He became Senior Vet there in 2011 and a Partner in 2013. He gained a GPCert(Ophthal) whilst in practice.

Sheldon's BSAVA career started immediately after graduation when he joined the East Anglia Regional Committee. He took on the roles of Treasurer, Secretary and Chair of the region and afterwards became a Regional Representative. This led him to be a committee member, and subsequently Chair of the Membership Development Committee. Sheldon became Honorary Treasurer of the Association in 2016.

A few notes on using this book

- Under the drug listings, only doses are mentioned; the more detailed information on contraindications, interactions, etc., can be found in the *BSAVA Small Animal Formulary*. This is to enable the information to be found quickly and to keep the bulk of the book down.
- Selected drugs are listed by generic name. (An index of trade names is provided at the back of the book.)
  - The rINN generic name is used.
  - The list of trade names is not necessarily comprehensive, and the mention or exclusion of any particular commercial product is not a recommendation or otherwise as to its value. Any omission of a product that is authorized for a particular small animal indication is purely accidental.
  - Products that are not authorized for veterinary use by the Veterinary Medicines Directorate are marked with an asterisk. Note that an indication that a product is authorized does not necessarily mean that it is authorized for all species and indications listed in the monograph; users should check individual datasheets.
- Drug doses are based on those recommended by the manufacturers in their datasheets and package inserts, **or** are based on those given in published articles or textbooks, **or** are based on clinical experience. These recommendations should be used only as guidelines and should not be considered appropriate for every case. Clinical judgement must take precedence. Where possible, doses have been given for individual species; however, sometimes generalizations are used. 'Small mammals' includes ferrets, lagomorphs and rodents. 'Birds' includes psittacines, raptors, pigeons and others. 'Reptiles' includes chelonians, lizards and snakes. Except where indicated, all doses given for ectothermic animals (reptiles) assume that the animal is kept within its Preferred Optimum Temperature Zone (POTZ). Animals that are maintained at different temperatures may have different rates of metabolism and therefore the dose (and especially the frequency) that is required may require alteration. ⬛⬛⬛➡

- A veterinary surgeon should always refer to other source material if they are not familiar with the drugs mentioned in this guide.
- The tables of tablet sizes for various weights of animal are taken from the datasheets of certain authorized brands of the drug and are identified as such. Where several brands of the same drug use different sized tablets and have each produced a different table, only one has been included. If this is not the brand used in your clinic, I would encourage you to use the blank pages to personalize your guide.
- Likewise, an algorithm for suggested course of investigation of a certain disease should not be considered in isolation but should be used in context with the relevant Manual or other source material.
- All sources used in this guide are referenced by a superscript number which refers to a bibliography at the back of the book.

Abdomen – abdominocentesis [20]

Positioning and preparation

- Sedation may or may not be required.
- The dog should be restrained in right lateral recumbency and it might be worth emptying the patient's bladder before the procedure.
- The abdomen should be clipped and prepared as for a non-surgical procedure.

Equipment

A 5 ml syringe, collection tubes (EDTA, plain and sterile) and some microscope slides should be prepared.

Use an 18–22 G, 2.5–3.75 cm needle or over-the-needle catheter.

Technique

Abdominocentesis can be performed by a single centesis or using a four-quadrant approach.

1. The site for single abdominocentesis is a point 1 cm lateral and to the right of the ventral midline and 1–2 cm caudal to the umbilicus.
2. Once the needle has been inserted through the skin and abdominal wall, allow fluid to drip from the needle (or catheter with needle removed) into a tube, or gently aspirate with a 2–5 ml syringe. Unless there is a large volume of free fluid it is preferable to allow it to drip from the needle hub, rather than aspirating, to avoid sucking omentum or viscera into the needle.

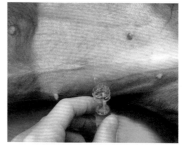

⸬⮕

3. If fluid is not obtained from the first site, repeat the procedure in the three remaining sites.

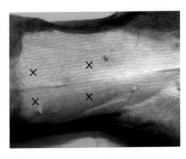

4. Collect fluid into an EDTA tube for cytology and cell count, and into a plain tube for culture and biochemical analysis.
5. Make several air-dried smears.

NOTES

NOTES

Abdominal swelling – diagnostic work-up[20]

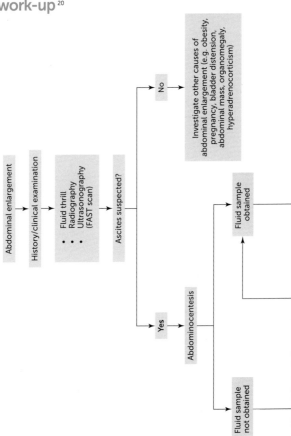

Abdominal enlargement → History/clinical examination →

- Fluid thrill
- Radiography
- Ultrasonography (FAST scan)

→ Ascites suspected?

No → Investigate other causes of abdominal enlargement (e.g. obesity, pregnancy, bladder distension, abdominal mass, organomegaly, hyperadrenocorticism)

Yes → Abdominocentesis → Fluid sample obtained

Fluid sample not obtained

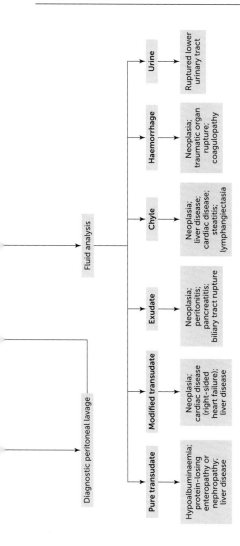

Diagnostic peritoneal lavage

Fluid analysis

Pure transudate
Hypoalbuminaemia; protein-losing enteropathy or nephropathy; liver disease

Modified transudate
Neoplasia; cardiac disease (right-sided heart failure); liver disease

Exudate
Neoplasia; peritonitis; pancreatitis; biliary tract rupture

Chyle
Neoplasia; liver disease; cardiac disease; steatitis; lymphangiectasia

Haemorrhage
Neoplasia; traumatic organ rupture; coagulopathy

Urine
Ruptured lower urinary tract

See also FAST scan – abdominal

Acepromazine (ACP) [25, 26]
(ACP) POM-V

Formulations:
- Injectable: 2 mg/ml solution.
- Oral: 10 mg, 25 mg tablets.

DOSES

Dogs (not Boxers), Cats: 0.01–0.02 mg/kg slowly i.v.;
0.01–0.05 mg/kg i.m., s.c.; 1–3 mg/kg p.o.
- Boxers: 0.005–0.01 mg/kg i.m.

Mammals:
- Primates (small): 0.5–1 mg/kg p.o.
- Marsupials: 0.2 mg/kg i.m., s.c., p.o.
- Ferrets: 0.2–0.5 mg/kg i.m., s.c., p.o.
- Rabbits: 0.1–1.0 mg/kg i.m., s.c.
- Guinea pigs: 0.5–5 mg/kg i.m., s.c., p.o.
- Hamsters: 0.5–5 mg/kg i.m., s.c., p.o.
- Gerbils: 3 mg/kg i.m., s.c., p.o.; reduces the seizure
  threshold in susceptible strains of gerbil and is not
  recommended
- Rats: 0.5–2.5 mg/kg i.m., s.c., p.o.
- Mice: 0.5–5 mg/kg i.m., s.c., p.o. The higher doses
  should only be given orally.

Birds: Not recommended.

Reptiles: 0.1–0.5 mg/kg i.m.

Amphibians, Fish: No information available.

See also Sedation combinations

NOTES

Acid–base disturbances – interpreting results [12]

Disorder	pH	pCO$_2$	Base excess	Bicarbonate
Metabolic acidosis	↓	(↓)	Negative	↓
Metabolic alkalosis	↑	(↑)	Positive	↑
Respiratory acidosis	↓	↑	(Positive)	(↑)
Respiratory alkalosis	↑	↓	(Negative)	(↓)

Acid–base disturbances – metabolic causes [12]

Metabolic acidosis

- High anion gap (normochloraemic)
- Diabetic *ketoacidosis*
- *Lactic acidosis*
- *Uraemic acidosis*
- Toxins (e.g. ethylene glycol, salicylates)
- Normal anion gap (hyperchloraemic)
- *Diarrhoea*
- Renal tubular acidosis
- Drugs (e.g. carbonic anhydrase inhibitors)
- Dilutional acidosis

Metabolic alkalosis

- Associated with hypochloraemia
- *Vomiting*
- *Diuretic therapy*
- Following hypercapnia
- Not typically associated with hypochloraemia
- Primary hyperaldosteronism
- Hyperadrenocorticism

Diagnoses in *italics* are those encountered most frequently in clinical practice.

Acid—base disturbances — respiratory causes [12]

Respiratory acidosis (hypoventilation)

- Upper airway obstruction
- Respiratory centre depression
- Central neurological disease
- Drugs, e.g. anaesthesia
- Neuromuscular disease, e.g. myasthenia gravis, polyradiculoneuritis, botulism
- Restrictive disease, e.g. pneumothorax, pleural effusion
- Respiratory muscle fatigue, e.g. severe parenchymal disease
- Inadequate mechanical ventilation

Respiratory alkalosis (hyperventilation)

- Hypoxaemia (severe)
- Pulmonary parenchymal disease
- Hyperthermia
- Pain
- Fear/stress
- Exercise
- Neurological disease
- Excessive mechanical ventilation

Activated charcoal *see* Charcoal

Adrenaline (Epinephrine) [25, 26]
(Adrenaline*, Epinephrine*) POM

Formulations: Injectable: Range of concentrations for injection: 0.1–10 mg/ml, equivalent to 1:10,000 to 1:100.

DOSES

Dogs, Cats:

■ Cardiopulmonary arrest (CPA): 10 µg (micrograms)/kg of a 1:1000 solution (1000 µg/ml) given i.v. or intraosseously every 3–5 minutes. Peripheral administration into a vein should be followed by a fluid bolus to push the drug into the central circulation. High dose epinephrine (0.1 mg/kg i.v.) may be considered after prolonged CPA. Can be given intratracheally for

resuscitation of intubated animals, but higher doses may be required. A long catheter should be used to ensure the drug is delivered into the bronchi beyond the end of the endotracheal tube
- Bronchoconstriction and anaphylaxis: 10 µg (micrograms)/kg of a 1:1000 solution (1000 µg/ml) i.v. or i.m. The i.v. route is preferred if hypotension accompanies an anaphylactoid reaction.

Mammals:
- Ferrets: 20 µg (micrograms)/kg s.c., i.m., i.v., intratracheal
- Rabbits: cardiac resuscitation: 100 µg (micrograms)/kg i.v., repeated and/or higher doses (up to 200 µg/kg) may be required at intervals of 2–5 min
- Guinea pigs: 3 µg (micrograms)/kg i.v.
- Other rodents: 10 µg (micrograms)/kg i.v. as required.

Birds: 0.1–1.0 mg/kg i.m., i.v., intraosseous, intracardiac, intratracheal.

Reptiles: 0.5 mg/kg i.v., intraosseous; 1 mg/kg intratracheal diluted in 1 ml/100 g bodyweight.

Amphibians: No information available.

Fish: 0.2–0.5 mg/kg i.m., i.v., intraperitoneal, intracardiac.

Amitriptyline [25, 26]
(Amitriptyline*) POM

Formulations: Oral: 10 mg, 25 mg, 50 mg tablets; 5 mg/ml, 10 mg/ml solutions.

DOSES

Dogs: 1–2 mg/kg p.o. q12–24h.

Cats: 0.5–1 mg/kg p.o. q24h.

Mammals: Rats: 5–20 mg/kg p.o. q24h.

Birds: 1–2 mg/kg p.o. q12–24h; can be increased to 5 mg/kg if needed.

Reptiles, Amphibians, Fish: No information available.

Amlodipine [25]

(Amodip, Amlodipine*, Istin*) POM-V, POM

Formulations: Oral: 1.25 mg (cats), 5 mg, 10 mg tablets, 1 mg/ml and 2 mg/ml oral sugar-free solution.

DOSES

Dogs: Initial dose 0.05–0.1 mg/kg p.o. q12–24h. The dose may be titrated upwards weekly as required, up to 0.4 mg/kg, monitoring blood pressure regularly.

Cats: 0.625–1.25 mg/cat p.o. q24h. The dose may be increased slowly or the frequency increased to q12h if necessary. Blood pressure monitoring is essential.

Amodip (from datasheet)		
Dose rate (initial dose)	Patient bodyweight (kg)	No. of tablets per dose
Cats		
0.125–0.25 mg/kg q24h	2.5–5.0	0.5
	5.1–10.0	1
	>10	2

NOTES

Amoxicillin (Amoxycillin) [25, 26]

(Amoxibactin, Amoxycare, Amoxypen, Betamox, Bimoxyl, Clamoxyl) POM-V

Formulations:

- Injectable: 150 mg/ml suspension.
- Oral: 40 mg, 50 mg, 200 mg, 250 mg, 500 mg tablets; suspension which when reconstituted provides 50 mg/ml.
- Topical: 100% w/w powder for top dressing (Vetremox).

DOSES

Dogs, Cats:

- Parenteral: 7 mg/kg i.m. q24h; 15 mg/kg i.m. q48h for depot preparations
- Oral: 10 mg/kg p.o. q8–12h (doses of 16–33 mg/kg i.v. q8h are used in humans to treat serious infections).

Dose chosen will depend on site of infection, causal organism and severity of the disease.

Amoxibactin tablets (from datasheet)			
Patient bodyweight (kg)	**No. of tablets per dose, twice daily**		
	50 mg	*250 mg*	*500 mg*
Dogs and cats			
1–1.25	¼		
> 1.25–2.5	½		
> 2.5–3.75	¾		
> 3.75–5	1		
> 5–6.25	1¼		
Dogs			
> 5–6.25		¼	
> 6.25–12.5		½	¼
> 12.5–18.75		¾	
> 18.75–25		1	½

Amoxibactin tablets (from datasheet)			
Patient bodyweight (kg)	**No. of tablets per dose, twice daily**		
	50 mg	*250 mg*	*500 mg*
Dogs continued			
> 25–31.25		1¼	
> 31.25–37.5		1½	¾
> 37.5–50		2	1
> 50–62.5			1¼
> 62.5–75			1½

Mammals:

- Primates: 11 mg/kg p.o. q12h or 11 mg/kg s.c., i.m. q24h
- Sugar gliders: 30 mg/kg p.o., i.m. q24h for 14 days (for dermatitis)
- Hedgehogs: 15 mg/kg p.o., s.c., i.m. q8–12h
- Ferrets: 10–30 mg/kg s.c., p.o. q12h
- Rabbits: 7 mg/kg s.c. q24h
- Rats, Mice: 100–150 mg/kg i.m., s.c. q12h.

Birds: 150–175 mg/kg i.m., s.c. q8–12h (q24h for long-acting preparations)

- Raptors, Parrots: 175 mg/kg p.o. q12h
- Pigeons: 1–1.5 g/l drinking water (Vetremox pigeon) q24h for 3–5 days or 100–200 mg/kg p.o. q6–8h
- Waterfowl: 1 g/l drinking water (Amoxinsol soluble powder) alternate days for 3–5 days or 300–500 mg/kg p.o. (in soft food) for 3–5 days
- Passerines: 1.5 g/l drinking water for 3–5 days (Vetremox pigeon).

Reptiles: 5–10 mg/kg i.m., p.o. q12–24h (most species)

- Chelonians: 5–50 mg/kg i.m., p.o. q12h.

Amphibians: No information available.

Fish: 40–80 mg/kg in feed q24h for 10 days or 12.5 mg/kg i.m. once (long-acting preparation).

Amoxicillin/Clavulanate *see* Co-amoxiclav

Ampicillin [25, 26]
(Amfipen, Ampicare) POM-V

Formulations:

- Injectable: Ampicillin sodium 250 mg, 500 mg powders for reconstitution (human licensed product only); 100 mg/ml long-acting preparation.
- Oral: 500 mg tablets; 250 mg capsule.

DOSES

Dogs:

- Routine infections: 10–20 mg/kg i.v., i.m., s.c., p.o. q6–8h
- CNS or serious bacterial infections: up to 40 mg/kg i.v. q6h has been recommended.

Cats: 10–20 mg/kg i.v., i.m., s.c., p.o. q6–8h.

Mammals:

- Primates: 20 mg/kg p.o., i.m., i.v. q8h
- Ferrets: 5–30 mg/kg i.m., s.c. q12h
- Gerbils: 20–100 mg/kg s.c. q8h or 6–30 mg/kg p.o. q8h
- Rats, Mice: 25 mg/kg i.m., s.c. q12h or 50–200 mg/kg p.o. q12h
- Rabbits, Chinchillas, Guinea pigs, Hamsters: do not use.

Birds: 50–100 mg/kg i.v., i.m. q8–12h, 150–200 mg/kg p.o. q8–12h, 1–2 g/l drinking water, 2–3 g/kg in soft feed.

Reptiles: 10–20 mg/kg s.c., i.m. q24h (most species)

- Hermann's tortoises: 50 mg/kg i.m. q12h.

Amphibians: No information available.

Fish: 50–80 mg/kg in feed q24h for 10 days.

Anaphylaxis – emergency treatment [5]

Identification

Anaphylaxis is an acute severe allergic reaction characterized by venous and arteriolar dilation and increased capillary permeability, which, in severe cases, result in decreased venous return to the heart, hypotension and hypoperfusion. Signs of anaphylaxis include:

- Angioedema: this commonly results in swelling of the face and distal limbs, but can include swelling of the pharynx and larynx
- Bronchospasm
- Pruritus
- Urticaria: raised red skin wheals or hives
- Vomiting
- Anaphylactic shock.

Procedure

1. Perform a rapid assessment of the airway, respiration and circulation.
2. If upper airway obstruction is evident with spontaneous respiration:
   - Perform endotracheal (ET) intubation with sedation as required
   - Administer supplemental oxygen as required: if measurements of oxygen are unavailable administer 100% oxygen.
3. Establish vascular access.
4. In life-threatening cases with evidence of upper airway obstruction or cardiovascular collapse (hypotension, bradycardia), give 0.02 mg/kg adrenaline i.v. slowly. *(Adrenaline can be given into the trachea if intravenous access is difficult, but may be ineffective. Insert a dog urinary catheter via the ET tube to the level of the carina. Dilute adrenaline with saline or sterile water.)*
   - Initiate monitoring of ECG, S_pO_2, $ETCO_2$, blood pressure, venous blood gas, acid–base and electrolyte status.

- Monitor for adrenaline-induced arrhythmias and hypertension.

5. Treat hypoperfusion with intravenous fluid therapy and vasopressors as required.
   - Crystalloids should be administered in boluses, as required, to achieve normotension (mean arterial pressure of 80–120 mmHg, systolic arterial pressure of 100–200 mmHg) and good perfusion (lactate <2.5 mmol/l).
   - Vasopressors, such as dobutamine (5–15 µg (micrograms)/kg/min) or dopamine (3–10 µg/kg/min), should be considered if hypotension is unresponsive to fluid therapy.

6. Following initial emergency treatment, if bronchospasm and angioedema persist, consider dexamethasone (0.5 mg/kg i.v. once).

7. Long-term prophylaxis requires identification and avoidance of the causative agent.

NOTES

Anorexia in rabbits – an approach to evaluation [23]

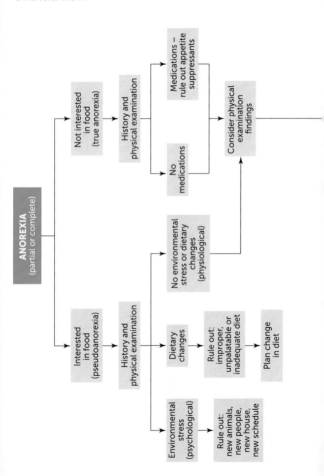

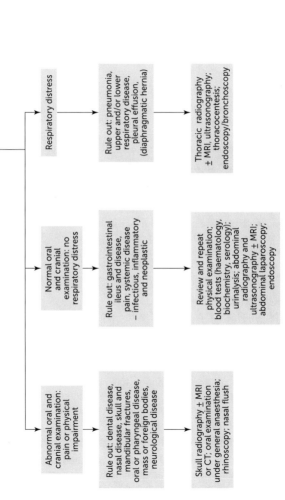

Anticoagulant rodenticide poisoning (CAUTION) [1]

Also known as: Brodifacoum, bromadiolone, chlorophacinone, coumatetralyl, difenacoum, diphacinone, flocoumafen, warfarin

Description/exposure

Anticoagulant rodenticide (ACR) exposure occurs by ingestion of rodenticide bait products. Cats are more resistant to ACR than dogs. Relay toxicosis (secondary to ingestion of poisoned mice) is rare in dogs and cats.

Mechanism of action

ACRs act by blocking the conversion of inactive, oxidized vitamin K to its active, reduced form (vitamin K hydroquinone). When active vitamin K is depleted, the liver is unable to activate coagulation factors II, VII, IX, and X, resulting in a life-threatening coagulopathy. Cavitary bleeding, as well as bleeding into the pulmonary parenchyma, pericardium, gastrointestinal tract, skin and from the nasal mucosa are some sequelae of coagulopathy.

Clinical presentation

The time from exposure to the development of clinical signs is typically 3–5 days, thus patients acutely exposed to rodenticide (<24–36 hours) may present without clinical signs or evidence of coagulopathy. Those presenting with clinical signs typically show evidence of coagulopathy and haemorrhagic shock. Dyspnoea, haemoptysis, tachycardia, pallor, poor pulse quality, tachypnoea and altered mentation are commonly seen. Melena, epistaxis, petechiae, bleeding from the gums and ecchymoses are less common.

Diagnostics

The prothrombin time (PT) should be measured to assess the degree of coagulopathy. Factor VII has the shortest half-life (6.2 hours) of the vitamin K-dependent coagulation factors and depletion is seen within approximately 36–48 hours.

Evaluation of the extrinsic coagulation pathway through PT evaluation confirms a toxic dose of ACR. A prolonged PT is a typical finding with clinical evidence of bleeding. Routine blood work (haematology and serum chemistry) should be evaluated for anaemia and to rule out other causes of coagulopathy (e.g. thrombocytopenia). Whole blood and gastric contents can be submitted for confirmation of the presence of ACR, if indicated; however, results are often delayed for several days, and treatment should not be withheld in a clinically symptomatic patient. Radiography and ultrasonography (especially focused assessment with sonography for trauma or 'FAST scans') should be considered to look for evidence of cavitary bleeding (e.g. pleural effusion, pericardial effusion, abdominal effusion).

Treatment

Patients recently exposed to ACR should undergo gastrointestinal decontamination, typically with the induction of emesis and administration of one dose of activated charcoal. A one-time injection of vitamin K1 should be avoided, as this alters the results of the PT 48 hours post-exposure. In the acutely poisoned ACR patient, fluid therapy, hospitalization and supportive care in a hospital environment are not necessary. Approximately 36–48 hours post-exposure, the PT should be reassessed; if it is within normal limits, non-toxic levels were achieved. However, if the PT is prolonged, prompt therapy with oral vitamin K1 is warranted (3–5 mg/kg divided q12h for 30 days). The PT should be rechecked 48 hours after the last dose of oral vitamin K1 (approximately day 32); if prolonged, an additional 2 weeks of therapy is warranted.

If the patient presents with bleeding due to a coagulopathy, treatment with fresh frozen plasma (FFP) or frozen plasma (FP) is warranted to replace the clotting factors. Vitamin K1 alone is not curative, as normalization of the PT takes approximately 12 hours following the initiation of therapy, therefore patients with an acute coagulopathy require factor replacement. Supportive care in the form ⟶

of oxygen therapy, crystalloid fluids, plasma transfusions
and even whole blood transfusions may be necessary.
Concurrent treatment with vitamin K1 for 30 days should be
initiated. When administering vitamin K1, ideally oral rather
than parenteral administration should occur due to the rapid
absorption from the gastrointestinal tract.

Prognosis

Early decontamination and treatment is associated with an
excellent prognosis. Clinically bleeding patients also
have an excellent prognosis if treatment is immediate
and appropriate.

NOTES

Apomorphine [25, 26]
(Apometic) POM-V

Formulations: Injectable: 10 mg/ml solution in 2 ml or 5 ml ampoules; 5 mg/ml, 10 mg/ml solutions in 10 ml pre-filled syringes. Other non-authorized formulations available.

DOSES

Dogs: 0.2 mg/kg s.c. (authorized dose), 20–40 µg (micrograms)/kg i.v. (non-authorized dose and route but some evidence to suggest is at least as effective).

Apometic 10 mg/ml (from datasheet)		
Dose rate	Patient bodyweight (kg)	Volume required (ml)
Dogs		
0.2 mg/kg	5	0.10
	10	0.20
	15	0.30
	20	0.40
	25	0.50
	30	0.60
	35	0.70
	40	0.80
	45	0.90
	50	1.00

Cats: Not recommended; xylazine is a potent emetic in cats and at least as safe.

Mammals: Ferrets: 70 µg (micrograms)/kg s.c.

Birds, Reptiles, Amphibians, Fish: No information available.

Arterial thromboembolism key points [12]

- Typical clinical signs: acute onset, often no previous history of a cardiac disease, hindlimbs more frequently affected than forelimbs, five 'Ps' – paralysis/paresis, pain, pulselessness, pallor (or cyanotic nail beds and footpads), polar (cold distal limbs and footpads). Cats are frequently tachypnoeic or may even show open-mouth breathing. In dogs, arterial thrombosis has generally a more chronic progression and is not associated with cardiac disease.

- Diagnosis: physical examination findings are highly suggestive of arterial thromboembolism (ATE). On urgent standing echocardiogram and electrocardiogram (U-SEE) examination, a right parasternal long-axis or right parasternal short-axis view typically reveals an enlarged left atrium in cats and 'smoke' or a thrombus may additionally be present. Such findings are consistent with cardiogenic ATE. Tachypnoea/dyspnoea is frequently caused by stress and pain, and not necessarily pulmonary oedema. Thoracic radiographs should be obtained to confirm the presence of pulmonary oedema.

- Differential diagnoses: trauma, neurological diseases (e.g. brachial plexus avulsion, intervertebral disc extrusion).

- Treatment: opioid analgesia is the first priority, followed by anticoagulation therapy and congestive heart failure therapy (if pulmonary oedema is present).

- Prognosis: factors associated with a poor prognosis include bilateral rear limb involvement, no motor activity and hypothermia (<37.2°C).

NOTES

ASA physical status and classifications scale [7]

ASA scale	Physical description	Veterinary patient examples
1	Normal patient with no disease	Healthy patient scheduled for ovariohysterectomy or castration
2	Patient with mild systemic disease that does not limit normal function	Controlled diabetes mellitus, mild cardiac valve insufficiency
3	Patient with moderate systemic disease that limits normal function	Uncontrolled diabetes mellitus, symptomatic heart disease
4	Patient with severe systemic disease that is a constant threat to life	Sepsis, organ failure, heart failure
5	Patient that is moribund and not expected to live 24 hours without surgery	Shock, multiple organ failure, severe trauma
E	Describes patient as an emergency	Gastric dilatation–volvulus, respiratory distress

NOTES

Aspirin (Acetylsalicylic acid) [25, 26]

(Aspirin BP* and component of many others) P

Formulations: Oral: 75 mg, 300 mg tablets.

DOSES

Dogs: Doses are anecdotal and the ideal doses are unknown. For reduction of platelet aggregation doses of 0.5–1 mg/kg p.o. q24h and for analgesia/antipyretic/anti-inflammatory range from 10–20 mg/kg p.o. q12h. The safety and efficacy of this dose has not been established. Ultralow dose used in IMHA is 0.5 mg/kg p.o. q12h.

Cats: For reduction of platelet aggregation doses of ¼ of a 75 mg tablet (18.75 mg) p.o. for an average sized cat 3 days a week (low dose) or, alternatively, 75 mg for an average sized cat 3 days a week (high-dose); this dose may be associated with a higher risk of GI side effects. Some authors suggest a very low dose (0.5 mg/kg p.o. q24h) to inhibit platelet COX without preventing the beneficial effects of prostacyclin production. The safety and efficacy of these different doses have not been evaluated in clinical or experimental studies.

Mammals:
- Primates: 5–10 mg/kg p.o. q4–6h
- Ferrets: 10–20 mg/kg p.o. q24h
- Rabbits: 100 mg/kg p.o. q12–24h
- Rodents: 50–150 mg/kg p.o. q4–8h.

Birds: Parrots: 5 mg/kg p.o. q8h.

Reptiles, Amphibians, Fish: No information available.

Atipamezole [25, 26]

(Alzane, Antisedan, Atipam, Revertor, Sedastop, Tipafar)
POM-V

Formulations: Injectable: 5 mg/ml solution.

DOSES

Dogs:
- Five times the previous medetomidine dose or 10 times the previous dose of dexmedetomidine (0.5 mg/ml

solution) i.m. (i.e. equal volume of solution to medetomidine or dexmedetomidine 0.5 mg/ml solution given. The atipamezole dose in millilitres is one fifth ($\frac{1}{5}$) of the dose volume of dexmedetomidine 0.1 mg/ml solution. When medetomidine or dexmedetomidine has been administered at least an hour before, the dose of atipamezole can be reduced by half and repeated if recovery is slow

- Amitraz toxicity: 25 µg (micrograms)/kg i.m. but if there is no benefit within half an hour this can be repeated or incrementally increased every 30 minutes up to 200 µg/kg.

Cats: Two and a half times the previous medetomidine or five times the previous dose of dexmedetomidine (0.5 mg/ml solution) i.m. (i.e. half the volume of medetomidine or dexmedetomidine 0.5 mg/ml solution given. The atipamezole dose in millilitres is one tenth ($\frac{1}{10}$) of the dose volume of dexmedetomidine 0.1 mg/ml solution). When medetomidine or dexmedetomidine has been administered at least an hour before, the dose of atipamezole can be reduced by half and repeated if recovery is slow.

Mammals:

- Primates, Hedgehogs, Ferrets, Rodents: Five times the previous medetomidine dose s.c., i.m.
- Marsupials, Rabbits: Two and a half times the previous medetomidine dose. When medetomidine or dexmedetomidine has been administered at least an hour before, dose of atipamezole can be reduced by half (i.e. half the volume of medetomidine or dexmedetomidine) and repeated if recovery is slow
- Amitraz toxicity: 25 µg (micrograms)/kg i.m. but if there is no benefit within half an hour this can be repeated or incrementally increased every 30 minutes up to 200 µg/kg.

Birds, Reptiles: Two and a half to five times the previous medetomidine or dexmedetomidine dose i.m., i.v.

Amphibians, Fish: No information available.

Azotaemia differentiation [12]

Parameter	Pre-renal (intrinsic)	Renal	Post-renal
Urine specific gravity	Hypersthenuric (>1.040 in cats and >1.030 in dogs) unless complicating disease is present, e.g. hypoadrenocorticism, hypercalcaemia, *Escherichia coli* sepsis	Variable depending on stage of disease but often isosthenuric (1.008–1.012) or poorly concentrated (<1.025)	Variable
Dipstick results	Generally unremarkable	Glucosuria and proteinuria common	
Sediment examination	Generally unremarkable	Casts, erythrocytes, bacteria, leucocytes and/or neoplastic cells may be seen	Erythrocytes common
Bladder size	Generally small	Variable depending on stage of disease process	Either large and tense or absent
Diagnostic imaging	Kidneys and urinary tract unremarkable	Renomegaly and ultrasonographic changes possible. Small kidneys seen if the azotaemia is chronic	Possible abnormalities include: • Reno-, uretero-, cysto- or urethroliths • Ureteral dilatation • Free abdominal fluid • Contrast studies may reveal urinary tract rupture or obstruction

NOTES

Benazepril [25, 26]

(Benefortin, Cardalis, Fortekor, Fortekor-Plus, Nelio, Prilben, Vetpril, Kelapril) POM-V

Formulations: Oral: 2.5 mg, 5 mg, 20 mg tablets. Available in a compound preparation with spironolactone (Cardalis tablets) in the following formulations: 2.5 mg benazepril/20 mg spironolactone, 5 mg benazepril/40 mg spironolactone, 10 mg benazepril/80 mg spironolactone. Also available in compound preparation with pimobendan (Fortekor Plus) in the following formulations, 1.25 mg pimobendan/2.5 mg benazepril, 5 mg pimobendan/10 mg benazepril.

DOSES

Dogs: Heart failure: 0.25–0.5 mg/kg p.o. q24h. For adjunctive treatment of hypotension/proteinuria 0.25–0.5 mg/kg p.o. q12–24h.

Cats: Chronic renal insufficiency: 0.5–1.0 mg/kg p.o. q24h. For adjunctive therapy in heart failure 0.25–0.5 mg/kg p.o. q24h.

Fortekor (from datasheet)							
Dose rate	**Patient bodyweight (kg)**	**No. of tablets required**					
		2.5 mg		**5 mg**		**20 mg**	
		SD	*DD*	*SD*	*DD*	*SD*	*DD*
Dogs							
0.25–0.5 mg/kg q24h	2.5–<5	0.5	1				
	5–10	1	2	0.5	1		
	11–20			1	2		
	21–40					0.5	1
	41–80					1	2
Cats							
0.5–1.0 mg/kg q24h	2.5–5	1					
	>5–10	2					

DD = double dose; SD = standard dose.

Mammals:
- Ferrets: 0.25–0.5 mg/kg p.o. q24h
- Rabbits, Guinea pigs: starting dose 0.05 mg/kg p.o. q24h. Dose may be increased to a maximum of 0.1 mg/kg
- Rats: anecdotally, ACE inhibitors have been used to mitigate protein-losing nephropathy in rats at 0.5–1.0 mg/kg p.o. q24h.

Birds, Reptiles, Amphibians, Fish: No information available.

NOTES

Blood glucose in rabbits [23]

Blood glucose concentration (mmol/l)	Significance	Possible reasons	Comments
<2	Severely hypoglycaemic	Insulinoma; paraneoplastic syndrome; artifact; metabolic disease; pancreatitis	Further investigations and repeat blood samples are necessary
2–4.1	Moderately hypoglycaemic	Lack of food	Often a feature of early gastrointestinal hypomotility and insufficient uptake of glucose and its precursors from the gut
4.2–8.2	Within reference range	N/a	Reassuring
8.3–12	Within normal range for pet rabbits that have been transported to unfamiliar surroundings	Mild stress	Reassuring but indicative that the rabbit is stressed; if other signs (anorexia, abdominal pain, suspected gastric dilation) are present then resampling is indicated
12.1–15	Slightly hyperglycaemic	Stress	Probably stress-induced but could be start of serious disease; resample unless clinical signs resolve rapidly

15.1–20	Significantly hyperglycaemic	Stress; pain	Possibly but not definitely surgical; resample after 30–60 minutes; take radiographs
20.1–25	Severely hyperglycaemic	Severe pain; deranged glucose metabolism	Serious disease is present; needs a diagnosis and surgery is likely; exploratory laparotomy is indicated, unless gas can be seen in the caecum indicating that an intestinal foreign body has passed through; monitoring and supportive care are essential
>25	Critically hyperglycaemic or diabetic	Severe pain; deranged glucose metabolism	If rabbit is ill, its condition is probably surgical or terminal; other findings from clinical examination and radiography need to be examined as well; if the rabbit is eating well, the possibility of diabetes needs to be investigated

Blood pressure *see* Hypertension

Body condition scoring scheme – cats [29]

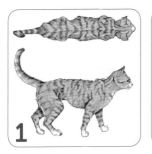

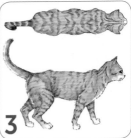

Under ideal

1 Ribs visible on shorthaired cats. No palpable fat. Severe abdominal tuck. Lumbar vertebrae and wings of ilia easily palpated.

2 Ribs easily visible on shorthaired cats. Lumbar vertebrae obvious. Pronounced abdominal tuck. No palpable fat.

3 Ribs easily palpable with minimal fat covering. Lumbar vertebrae obvious. Obvious waist behind ribs. Minimal abdominal fat.

Ideal

4 Ribs palpable with minimal fat covering. Noticeable waist behind ribs. Slight abdominal tuck. Abdominal fat pad absent.

5 Well-proportioned. Observe waist behind ribs. Ribs palpable with slight fat covering. Abdominal fat pad minimal.

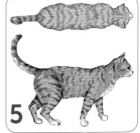

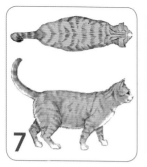
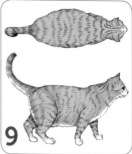

Over ideal

6 Ribs palpable with slight excess fat covering. Waist and abdominal fat pad distinguishable but not obvious. Abdominal tuck absent.

7 Ribs not easily palpated with moderate fat covering. Waist poorly discernible. Obvious rounding of abdomen. Moderate abdominal fat pad.

8 Ribs not palpable with excess fat covering. Waist absent. Obvious rounding of abdomen with prominent abdominal fat pad. Fat deposits present over lumbar area.

9 Ribs not palpable under heavy fat cover. Heavy fat deposits over lumbar area, face and limbs. Distention of abdomen with no waist. Extensive abdominal fat deposits.

Courtesy of WSAVA Global Nutrition Committee

NOTES

Body condition scoring scheme — dogs [29]

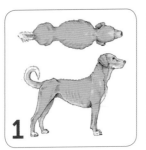

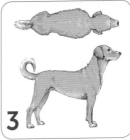

Under ideal

1 Ribs, lumbar vertebrae, pelvic bones and all bony prominences evident from a distance. No discernible body fat. Obvious loss of muscle mass.

2 Ribs, lumbar vertebrae and pelvic bones easily visible. No palpable fat. Some evidence of other bony prominences. Minimal loss of muscle mass.

3 Ribs easily palpated and maybe visible with no palpable fat. Tops of lumbar vertebrae visible. Pelvic bones becoming prominent. Obvious waist and abdominal tuck.

Ideal

4 Ribs easily palpable, with minimal fat covering. Waist easily noted, viewed from above. Abdominal tuck evident.

5 Ribs palpable without excess fat covering. Waist observed behind ribs when viewed from above. Abdomen tucked up when viewed from side.

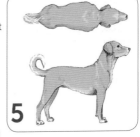

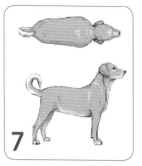
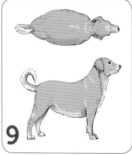

Over ideal

6 Ribs palpable with slight excess fat covering. Waist is discernible viewed from above but is not prominent. Abdominal tuck apparent.

7 Ribs palpable with difficulty; heavy fat cover. Noticeable fat deposits over lumbar area and base of tail. Waist absent or barely visible. Abdominal tuck may be present.

8 Ribs not palpable under very heavy fat cover, or palpable only with significant pressure. Heavy fat deposits over lumbar area and base of tail. Waist absent. No abdominal tuck. Obvious abdominal distention may be present.

9 Massive fat deposits over thorax, spine and base of tail. Waist and abdominal tuck absent. Fat deposits on neck and limbs. Obvious abdominal distention.

Courtesy of WSAVA Global Nutrition Committee

NOTES

Bodyweight (BW) to body surface area (BSA) conversion tables [25]

Dogs
(Formula: BSA (m^2) = 0.101 × (bodyweight in kg)$^{2/3}$)

BW (kg)	BSA (m^2)
0.5	0.06
1	0.1
2	0.16
3	0.21
4	0.25
5	0.3
6	0.33
7	0.37
8	0.4
9	0.44
10	0.47
11	0.5
12	0.53
13	0.56
14	0.59
15	0.61
16	0.64
17	0.67
18	0.69
19	0.72
20	0.74
22	0.79
24	0.84

BW (kg)	BSA (m^2)
26	0.89
28	0.93
30	0.98
35	1.08
40	1.18
45	1.28
50	1.37
55	1.46
60	1.55

Cats
(Formula: BSA (m^2) = 0.1 × (bodyweight in kg)$^{2/3}$)

BW (kg)	BSA (m^2)
0.5	0.06
1	0.1
1.5	0.134
2	0.163
2.5	0.184
3	0.208
3.5	0.231
4	0.252
4.5	0.273
5	0.292
5.5	0.316
6	0.33

Bromhexine [25, 26]
(Bisolvon) POM-V

Formulations:
- Injectable: 3 mg/ml solution.
- Oral: 10 mg/g powder.

DOSES

Dogs: Mucolysis: 3–15 mg/dog i.m. q12h; 2 mg/kg p.o. q12h.

Cats: Mucolysis: 3 mg/cat i.m. q24h; 1 mg/kg p.o. q24h.

Bisolvon (from datasheet)				
Dose of bromhexine HCl	Patient bodyweight (kg)	Dose of Bisolvon Powder (g)	No. of blue (0.5 g) scoops	Frequency and duration
Dogs				
2 mg/kg	5	0.5	1	Twice daily for 5 days
	15	1.5	3	
Cats				
1 mg/kg	5	0.5	1	Once daily for 7 days

Mammals: 0.3 mg/animal p.o. q24h or via nebulizer as 0.15 mg/ml for 20–30 minutes, 1–3 times daily.

Birds: 1.5 mg/kg i.m., p.o. q12–24h.

Reptiles: 0.1–0.2 mg/kg p.o. q24h.

Amphibians, Fish: No information available.

NOTES

Buprenorphine [25, 26]
(Bupaq, Buprecare, Buprenodale, Buprevet, Vetergesic)
POM-V CD SCHEDULE 3

Formulations: Injectable: 0.3 mg/ml solution; available in 1 ml vials that do not contain a preservative, or in 10 ml multidose bottle that contains chlorocresol as preservative.

DOSES

Dogs: Analgesia: 0.02 mg/kg i.v., i.m., s.c. q6h.

Cats: Analgesia: 0.02–0.03 mg/kg i.v., i.m., s.c. q6h. Also well tolerated and effective when given oral transmucosally.

Mammals: Analgesia:
- Ferrets: 0.01–0.10 mg/kg s.c., i.m., i.v q8–12h
- Rabbits: 0.03–0.06 mg/kg s.c., i.m., i.v q6–12h (doses <0.03 mg/kg have very limited analgesic effects but still have some sedative effects)
- Guinea pigs, Gerbils, Hamsters, Rats: 0.01–0.05 mg/kg i.m., s.c. q6–12h
- Mice: 0.05–0.1 mg/kg i.m., s.c. q6–12h.

 Anecdotally, oral transmucosal delivery appears effective in rabbits and chinchillas.

Birds: Analgesia: 0.01–0.05 mg/kg i.v., i.m q8–12h.
- African Grey Parrots: 0.25 mg/kg i.m. q8–12h.
- Chickens: 0.25–0.5 mg/kg i.m. q8–12h.

Reptiles: Analgesia: Doses of 0.01–0.1 mg/kg i.m. q24–48h have been suggested. Administration into the front limbs is recommended over the hind limbs for optimal systemic drug concentrations.

Amphibians:
- Leopard frog: 38 mg/kg s.c.
- Newt: 50 mg/kg intracoelomic q24h.

Fish: Analgesia: 0.01–0.1 mg/kg i.m

See also Sedation combinations

Butorphanol [25, 26]
(Alvegesic, Dolorex, Torbugesic, Torbutrol, Torphasol)
POM-V

Formulations:
- Injectable: 10 mg/ml solution.
- Oral: 5 mg, 10 mg tablets.

DOSES

Dogs:
- Analgesia: 0.2–0.5 mg/kg i.v., i.m., s.c.
- Antitussive: 0.05–0.1 mg/kg i.v., i.m., s.c., 0.5–1 mg/kg p.o q6–12h.

Cats: Analgesia: 0.2–0.5 mg/kg i.v., i.m., s.c.

Mammals: Analgesia:
- Primates: 0.01–0.02 mg/kg i.v., s.c., p.o. q4–6h
- Ferrets: 0.1–0.5 mg/kg s.c. q4–6h
- Rabbits: 0.1–0.5 mg/kg s.c q4h
- Chinchillas: 0.5–2 mg/kg s.c. q4h
- Guinea pigs: 0.2–2 mg/kg s.c. q4h
- Gerbils, Hamsters, Rats, Mice: 1–5 mg/kg s.c. q4h.

Birds: Analgesia: 0.3–4 mg/kg i.m., i.v. q6–12h.

Reptiles: Analgesia: Doses of 0.5–2 mg/kg i.m. q24h have been suggested.
- Bearded dragons, Green iguanas: 1.5 mg/kg i.m. q24h.

Amphibians:
- Leopard frog: 0.2–0.4 mg/kg i.m.
- Newt: 0.5 mg/l of water.

Fish: Analgesia: 0.25–5 mg i.m.
- Koi: 10 mg/kg i.m.

See also Sedation combinations

NOTES

NOTES

Cabergoline [25, 26]
(Galastop, Kelactin) POM-V

Formulations: Oral: 50 μg/ml solution.

DOSES

Dogs:
- 5 μg (micrograms)/kg p.o. q24h for 4–6 days. Control of aggression-related signs may require dosing for 2 weeks.
- To induce abortion: 15 μg (micrograms)/kg p.o. between days 30 and 42.

Cats: To induce abortion: 15 μg (micrograms)/kg p.o. between days 30 and 42.

Mammals: Rats: 10–50 μg (micrograms)/kg p.o. q12–24h or 600 μg/kg p.o. q72h for pituitary adenoma and associated mammary pathology.

Birds: 10–50 μg (micrograms)/kg p.o. q24h.

Reptiles, Amphibians, Fish: No information available.

Caffeine poisoning *see* Chocolate/caffeine poisoning

Carbimazole [25, 26]
(Vidalta) POM-V

Formulations: Oral: 10 mg, 15 mg tablets in a sustained release formulation.

DOSES

Dogs, Cats: Hyperthyroidism: starting dose 15 mg/animal p.o. q24h unless total thyroxine concentrations are <100 nmol/l in which case starting dose is 10 mg p.o. q24h. Adjust dose in 5 mg increments but do not break tablets.

Mammals: Guinea pigs: 1–2 mg/kg p.o. q24h.

Birds, Reptiles, Amphibians, Fish: No information available.

Cardiac silhouette *see* **Heart radiograph**

Cardiopulmonary resuscitation (CPR) [12]

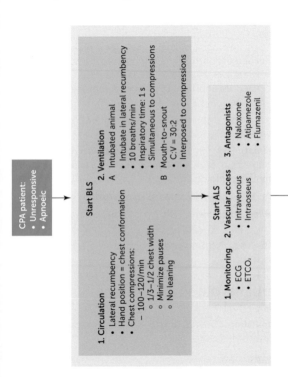

CPA patient:
• Unresponsive
• Apnoeic

Start BLS

1. Circulation
• Lateral recumbency
• Hand position = chest conformation
• Chest compressions:
  – 100–120/min
  ○ 1/3–1/2 chest width
  ○ Minimize pauses
  ○ No leaning

2. Ventilation
A Intubated animal
  • Intubate in lateral recumbency
  • 10 breaths/min
  • Inspiratory time: 1 s
  • Simultaneous to compressions
B Mouth-to-snout
  • C:V = 30:2
  • Interposed to compressions

Start ALS

1. Monitoring
• ECG
• ETCO$_2$

2. Vascular access
• Intravenous
• Intraosseus

3. Antagonists
• Naloxone
• Atipamezole
• Flumazenil

Basic life support (BLS) is started immediately after recognition of cardiopulmonary arrest (CPA), continued throughout the resuscitation effort and only interrupted every 2 minutes for short patient evaluations (electrocardiogram (ECG) and pulse). Advanced life support (ALS) measures occur whilst BLS is ongoing.

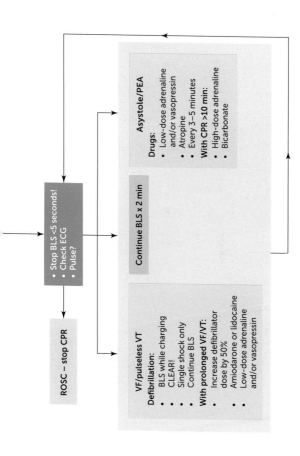

Stop BLS <5 seconds!
- Check ECG
- Pulse?

ROSC – stop CPR

Continue BLS x 2 min

Asystole/PEA

Drugs:
- Low-dose adrenaline and/or vasopressin
- Atropine
- Every 3–5 minutes

With CPR >10 min:
- High-dose adrenaline
- Bicarbonate

VF/pulseless VT

Defibrillation:
- BLS while charging
- CLEAR!
- Single shock only
- Continue BLS

With prolonged VF/VT:
- Increase defibrillator dose by 50%
- Amiodarone or lidocaine
- Low-dose adrenaline and/or vasopressin

C:V = compression:ventilation; ETCO$_2$ = end-tidal carbon dioxide; PEA = pulseless electrical activity; ROSC = return of spontaneous circulation; VF = ventricular fibrillation; VT = ventricular tachycardia.

Cardiopulmonary resuscitation – drugs [3]

Drug	Dose	Volume required according to bodyweight					
		5 kg	10 kg	20 kg	30 kg	40 kg	50 kg
Adrenaline (low-dose) 1:10000 (0.1 mg/ml)	0.01 mg/kg	0.5 ml	1 ml	2 ml	3 ml	4 ml	5 ml
Adrenaline (high-dose) 1:1000 (1 mg/ml)	0.1 mg/kg	0.5 ml	1 ml	2 ml	3 ml	4 ml	5 ml
Atropine (0.6 mg/ml)	0.04 mg/kg	0.3 ml	0.7 ml	1.4 ml	2.1 ml	2.8 ml	3.5 ml
Lidocaine (20 mg/ml)	2 mg/kg	0.5 ml	1 ml	2 ml	3 ml	4 ml	5 ml
Bicarbonate (1 mEq/ml)	1 mEq/kg	5 ml	10 ml	20 ml	30 ml	40 ml	50 ml

NOTES

Cardiovascular emergency sedation protocols [12]

Drug	Dosage	Comments
Light sedation		
Butorphanol (dogs and cats)	0.2–0.3 mg/kg i.v., i.m.	Short duration of sedation in anxious (but not fractious or aggressive) patients
Butorphanol (B) + acepromazine (ACP) (dogs)	0.2–0.3 mg/kg i.v., i.m. (B) + 0.01–0.02 mg/kg i.v., i.m. (ACP). Lower doses of ACP required in large-breed dogs and Boxers: 0.005–0.01 mg/kg i.v., i.m.	Needs relaxed period of time to work effectively
Butorphanol (B) + midazolam (M) (dogs)	0.2–0.3 mg/kg i.v., i.m. (B + M)	
Deeper sedation in cats		
Ketamine (K) + midazolam (M)	1.0–2.5 mg/kg i.v., p.o. (K) in severely fractious cats or 3.0–5.0 mg/kg i.m. (K) + 0.2–0.3 mg/kg i.v., i.m. (M)	Profound sedation lasting 15–20 minutes
Ketamine (K) + acepromazine (ACP) + butorphanol (B)	1.5 mg/kg i.v. (K) + 0.02 mg/kg i.m. (ACP) + 0.25 mg/kg i.m. (B)	Ketamine increases heart rate, which may be detrimental in cats with outflow tract obstruction and diastolic dysfunction
Butorphanol (B) + alfaxalone (A)	0.2 mg/kg i.m. (B) + 1.0–2.0 mg/kg i.m. (A)	Deep sedation useful for fractious or aggressive patients

Carprofen [25, 26]

(Canidryl, Carprodyl, Carprox Vet, Dolagis, Rimadyl, Rimifin)
POM-V

Formulations:

- Injectable: 50 mg/ml.
- Oral: 20 mg, 50 mg, 100 mg tablets (in plain and palatable formulations).

DOSES

Dogs: 4 mg/kg i.v., s.c. preoperatively or at time of anaesthetic induction; single dose should provide analgesia for up to 24 hours. Continued analgesia can be provided orally at 4 mg/kg/day, in single or divided dose for up to 5 days after injection. In dogs started on oral medication, subject to clinical response the dose may be reduced to 2 mg/kg/day, single dose, after 7 days.

Carprieve (from datasheet)			
Dose rate	Patient bodyweight (kg)	No. of tablets per dose	
		20 mg	*50 mg*
Dogs			
2 mg/kg once daily	5.0	½	
	10.0	1	
	12.5		½
	15.0	1½	
	20.0	2	
	25.0		1
	37.5		1½
	50.0		2

Cats: 4 mg/kg i.v., s.c., single dose preoperatively or at time of anaesthetic induction.

Mammals:
- Ferrets: 1–5 mg/kg total daily dose p.o.
- Rabbits: 2–4 mg/kg s.c. q24h or 1.5 mg/kg p.o. q24h
- Rodents: 2–5 mg/kg total daily dose i.v., i.m., s.c., p.o. in single or two divided doses
- Others: 2–4 mg/kg i.v., i.m., s.c. q24h.

Birds: 1–5 mg/kg i.m., s.c., p.o. q12–24h (higher rate appears effective for 24 hours). (Note: 3 mg/kg i.m. q12h was not sufficient to provide analgesia in experimentally induced arthritis.)

Reptiles: 4 mg/kg s.c., i.m., p.o. once, then 2 mg/kg s.c., i.m., p.o. q24h
- Bearded dragons: 2 mg/kg i.m. q24h.

Amphibians: No information available.

Fish: 1–5 mg/kg

Cascade *see* Prescribing cascade

NOTES

Cefalexin (Cephalexin) [25, 26]
(Cefaseptin, Cephacare, Cephorum, Ceporex, Rilexine, Therios, Tsefalen) POM-V

Formulations:
- Injectable: 180 mg/ml (18%) suspension.
- Oral: 50 mg, 75 mg, 120 mg, 250 mg, 300 mg, 500 mg, 600 mg, 750 mg, 1000 mg tablets; granules which, when reconstituted, provide a 100 mg/ml oral syrup.

DOSES

Dogs: 15 mg/kg p.o. q8–12h. Dose may be doubled in severe infections; 10 mg/kg i.m., s.c. q24h.

Cats: 15 mg/kg p.o. q8–12h; 10 mg/kg i.m., s.c. q24h.

Ceporex (from datasheet)				
Dose rate	Patient bodyweight (kg)	No. of tablets per dose, twice daily		
		50 mg	*250 mg*	*500 mg*
Dogs				
10–15 mg/kg twice daily for 5 days	≤5	1		
	6–9	2		
	10–25		1	
	26–50		2 or	1
	>51		3 or	2
Cats				
10–15 mg/kg twice daily for 5 days		1		

Mammals:
- Sugar gliders: 30 mg/kg s.c. q24h
- Hedgehogs: 25 mg/kg p.o. q8h
- Ferrets: 15–30 mg/kg p.o. q8–12h
- Rabbits: 15–20 mg/kg s.c. q12–24h

■ Guinea pigs: 25 mg/kg i.m. q12–24h.
■ Others: 15–30 mg/kg i.m. q8–12h.

Birds: 35–100 mg/kg p.o., i.m. q6–8h.

Reptiles: 20–40 mg/kg p.o. q12h.

Amphibians, Fish: No information available.

Cefovecin [25, 26]
(Convenia) POM-V

Formulations: Injectable: Lyophilized powder which when reconstituted contains 80 mg/ml cefovecin.

DOSES

Dogs, Cats: 8 mg/kg s.c., equivalent to 1 ml/10 kg of reconstituted drug subcutaneously. May be repeated after 14 days up to three times.

Convenia (from datasheet)		
Dose rate	**Patient bodyweight (kg)**	**Volume to be administered (ml)**
Dogs and cats		
8 mg/kg (additional doses administered 14 days after first injection)	2.5	0.25
	5	0.5
	10	1.0
	20	2.0
	40	4.0
	60	6.0

Mammals: Ferrets: 8 mg/kg s.c. every 2–3 days.

Birds, Reptiles: Initial data appear to show it is not practicable (half-life <2h in poultry and <4h in hens and green iguanas). Further data show that the half-life in parrots is similar to that in chickens.

Amphibians, Fish: No information available.

Charcoal (Activated charcoal) [25, 26, 27]

(Actidose-Aqua*, Charcodote*, Liqui-Char*) AVM-GSL

Formulations: Oral: 50 g activated charcoal (AC) powder or premixed slurry (200 mg/ml or 300 mg/ml available).

Administration:

- AC should be administered post emesis/gastric lavage; it acts as an adsorbent for many toxins and further reduces GI absorption.
- Slurries are more effective than tablets or capsules.
- Recommended dose is 1–4 g/kg and may be repeated every 4 to 6 hours for the first 24 to 48 hours or until charcoal is seen in the faeces.
- Repeat dose administration of AC is particularly important when the agent is enterohepatically recirculated, e.g. salicylates, barbiturates, theobromine and methylxanthines.
- AC slows GI transit time, thus co-administration of a cathartic (e.g. sorbitol or magnesium sulphate) can be considered although is not recommended in dehydrated patients or patients where there is a suspicion of ileus.
- AC use may be contraindicated if orally administered treatments or antidotes are to be given.

DOSES

Dogs, Cats: All uses: 0.5–4 g/kg p.o. as a slurry in water.

Mammals: 0.5–5 g/kg p.o. (anecdotal).

Birds: 50 ml/kg p.o.

Reptiles: Chelonians: 2–8 g/kg by stomach tube (anecdotal).

Amphibians, Fish: No information available.

NOTES

Chinchilla biological data [21]

Lifespan (years)	Average 8–10 (maximum 18)
Adult bodyweight (g)	Males: 450–600 Femal es: 550–800 (females are usually larger than males)
Dentition	2 [I 1/1, C0/0, P1/1, M3/3]
Body temperature (°C)	37–38
Heart rate (beats/min)	200–350
Respiratory rate (breaths/min)	40–80
Tidal volume (ml/kg)	Not found in the literature
Food consumption	21 g/day (adult); eat with fore feet
Water consumption	45–70 ml/day, depending on moisture content of food
Sexual maturity (months)	6–8
Oestrous cycle	40 days; seasonally polyoestrous (November to May)
Duration of oestrus	3–5 days
Gestation length (days)	111
Parturition	Early morning; does not usually nest
Post-partum oestrus	Yes
Litter size	1–6 (average 2)
Birth weight (g)	30–50; precocial; fully furred; active
Eyes open (days)	Open at birth
Eat solid food (days)	May begin day after birth to nibble solid foods
Weaning (days)	42
Litters per year	Produce 2 litters per year in captivity
Commercial breeding life	3 years, depending on culling rate
Chromosome number (diploid)	64

Chlorphenamine (Chlorpheniramine) [25, 26]
(Piriton*) POM, GSL

Formulations:
- Injectable: 10 mg/ml solution.
- Oral: 4 mg tablet, 0.4 mg/ml syrup.

DOSES

Dogs: Antihistamine: 4–8 mg/dog p.o. q8h; 2.5–10 mg/dog i.m. or slow i.v.

Cats: Antihistamine: 2–4 mg/cat p.o. q8–12h; 2–5 mg/cat i.m. or slow i.v.

Mammals:
- Primates: 0.5 mg/kg p.o. q24h
- Ferrets: 1–2 mg/kg p.o. q8–12h
- Rabbits: 0.2–0.4 mg/kg p.o. q12h
- Rodents: 0.6 mg/kg p.o. q24h.

Birds, Reptiles, Amphibians, Fish: No information available.

Chocolate/caffeine poisoning (URGENT) [1]
Also known as: methylxanthine, theobromine

Description/exposure

Chocolate is a very common toxicant in dogs that contains methylated xanthine alkaloids. Animals may also be exposed to other potentially dangerous sources of methylxanthines, including stimulants/caffeine pills, coffee grounds, coffee beans, energy drinks, weight loss supplements and body building supplements.

Mechanism of action

Methylxanthines work by inhibiting cellular phosphodiesterase (increasing cyclic adenosine monophosphate, cAMP), stimulating catecholamine release, increasing calcium entry into muscle cells and competitive inhibition of adenosine.

Clinical presentation

Clinical signs often include agitation, vomiting, diarrhoea, polyuria, polydipsia, tachycardia, arrhythmia (e.g. supraventricular tachycardia, ventricular premature complexes), ataxia, tremors and seizures. Death is possible at very high doses due to secondary complications (e.g. aspiration pneumonia).

Diagnostics

Blood work abnormalities seen with methylxanthines include hypokalaemia, hyperglycaemia and hypoglycaemia. Blood pressure measurement and electrocardiography are important monitoring and diagnostic tools in symptomatic patients.

Treatment

Aggressive gastrointestinal decontamination, including induction of emesis, is recommended. Chocolate can remain in the stomach for prolonged periods of time; therefore, emesis can be induced up to 6 hours following exposure. Gastric emptying should be considered with caution in patients that are already showing clinical signs (e.g. if neurologically inappropriate or cardiovascularly unstable). Multiple doses of activated charcoal without a cathartic should be given every 6 hours for 24 hours due to enterohepatic circulation. Intravenous fluids, anxiolytics (e.g. phenothiazines), beta-blockers, muscle relaxants and anticonvulsants may all be indicated depending on the severity of the clinical signs. Caffeine is absorbed by the bladder epithelium, so frequent walks to allow urination are important whilst hospitalized.

Prognosis

Excellent with supportive care.

Cimetidine [25, 26]

(Zitac, Cimetidine*, Dyspamet*, Tagamet*) POM-V, POM

Formulations:

- Injectable: 100 mg/ml solution in 2 ml ampoule.
- Oral: 100 mg, 200 mg, 400 mg, 800 mg tablets; 40 mg/ml syrup.

DOSES

Dogs: 5 mg/kg p.o., i.v., i.m. q8h.

Zitac (from datasheet)			
Dose rate (initial dose)	Patient bodyweight (kg)	No. of tablets per dose, three times daily	
		100 mg	*200 mg*
Dogs			
5 mg/kg q8h	6–10	½	
	11–20	1	½
	21–40		1
	41–60		1½

Cats: 2.5–5 mg/kg p.o., i.v., i.m. q12h.

Mammals:

- Primates: 10 mg/kg p.o., s.c., i.m. q8h
- Ferrets: 5–10 mg/kg i.m., s.c., p.o. q8h
- Rabbits: 5–10 mg/kg p.o. q6–8h
- Rodents: 5–10 mg/kg p.o., s.c., i.m., i.v. q6–12h.

Birds: 5 mg/kg i.m., p.o. q8–12h.

Reptiles: 4 mg/kg i.m., p.o. q8h.

Amphibians, Fish: No Information available.

NOTES

Clindamycin [25, 26]
(Antirobe, Clinacin, Clindacyl, Clindaseptin, Mycinor) POM-V

Formulations: Oral: 25 mg, 75 mg, 150 mg, 300 mg capsules and tablets; 25 mg/ml solution.

DOSES

Dogs: 5.5 mg/kg p.o. q12h or 11 mg/kg q24h; in severe infection can increase to 11 mg/kg q12h.
- Toxoplasmosis: 25 mg/kg p.o. daily in divided doses.

Cats: 5.5 mg/kg p.o. q12h or 11 mg/kg q24h.
- Toxoplasmosis: 25 mg/kg p.o. daily in divided doses.

Antirobe, Clindacin, Clindacyl (from datasheet)					
Dose rate	Patient bodyweight (kg)	No. of tablets required			
		25 mg	*75 mg*	*150 mg*	*300 mg*
Dogs and cats					
5.5 mg/kg q12h	4.5	1, twice daily			
	13.5		1, twice daily		
	27			1, twice daily	
11 mg/kg q24h	4.5	2, once daily			
	13.5			1, once daily	
	27				1, once daily
11 mg/kg q12h	4.5	2, twice daily			
	13.5			1, twice daily	
	27				1, twice daily

Mammals:
- Primates: 10 mg/kg p.o. q12h
- Sugar gliders, Hedgehogs: 5.5–10 mg/kg p.o. q12h
- Ferrets: 5.5–11 mg/kg p.o. q12h (toxoplasmosis: 12.5–25 mg/kg p.o. q12h)
- Rabbits, Rodents: *Do not use.*

Birds: 25 mg/kg p.o. q8h or 50 mg/kg p.o. q12h or 100 mg/kg p.o. q24h.
- Pigeons: 100 mg/kg p.o. q6h.

Reptiles: 2.5–5 mg/kg p.o. q24h.

Amphibians, Fish: No information available.

Co-amoxiclav (Amoxicillin/Clavulanate, Amoxycillin/Clavulanic acid) [25, 26]

(Clavabactin, Clavaseptin, Clavucill, Clavudale, Combimox, Combisyn, Kesium, Nisamox, Nisinject, Noroclav, Synuclav, Synulox, Twinox, Augmentin*) POM-V, POM

Formulations:
- Injectable: 175 mg/ml suspension (140 mg amoxicillin, 35 mg clavulanate); 600 mg powder (500 mg amoxicillin, 100 mg clavulanate); 1.2 g powder (1 g amoxicillin, 200 mg clavulanate) for reconstitution (Augmentin).
- Oral: 50 mg, 62.5 mg, 250 mg, 312.5 mg, 500 mg, 625 mg tablets each containing amoxicillin and clavulanate in a ratio of 4:1. Palatable drops which when reconstituted with water provide 40 mg amoxicillin and 10 mg clavulanic acid per ml. Note variation in labelling of products. The preparation size may be labelled in relation to amoxicillin quantity only or the combined amoxicillin clavulanic acid quantity.

DOSES

Dogs, Cats:
- Parenteral: 8.75 mg/kg (combined) i.v. q8h, i.m., s.c. q24h

- Oral: 12.5–25 mg/kg (combined) p.o. q8–12h.
  (Doses up to 25 mg/kg i.v. q8h are used to treat serious infections in humans.)

Clavucil, Synulox (from datasheet)			
Dose rate	Patient bodyweight (kg)	No. of tablets per dose, twice daily	
		50 mg	250 mg
Dogs and cats			
12.5 mg/kg q12h	1–2	½	
	3–5	1	
	6–9	2	
	10–13	3	
	14–18	4	
	19–25		1
	26–35		1½
	36–49		2
	50		3

Mammals:
- Primates: 15 mg/kg p.o. q24h
- Sugar gliders, Hedgehogs: 12.5 mg/kg p.o., s.c. q24h
- Ferrets: 12.5–20 mg/kg i.m., s.c. q12h
- Rats, Mice: 100 mg/kg p.o., s.c. q12h.

Birds: 125–150 mg/kg p.o., i.v. q12h; 125–150 mg/kg i.m. q24h.

Reptiles, Amphibians, Fish: No information available

NOTES

Codeine [25, 26]

(Pardale-V, Codeine*) POM

Formulations: Oral: 3 mg/5 ml paediatric linctus; 3 mg/ml linctus; 5 mg/ml syrup; 15 mg, 30 mg, 60 mg tablets.

DOSES

Dogs: General use: 0.5–2 mg/kg p.o. q12h. Do not use Pardale-V for codeine at this dose rate.

Cats: General use: 0.5–2 mg/kg p.o. q12h. Do not use formulation with paracetamol.

Amphibians: 42–53 mg/kg s.c. shown to provide analgesia for >4 h.

Mammals, Birds, Reptiles, Fish: No information available.

NOTES

Collapse [15]

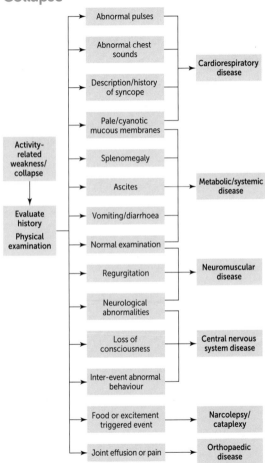

An approach to the work-up of animals with episodic weakness and collapse.

Congestive heart failure – acute stabilization [12]

The recommendations for acute stabilization (ACVIM Consensus Statement 2009) include:

- Hospitalization for cage rest and close monitoring (in a quiet, minimum stress environment where possible)
- Oxygen therapy
- Opioid sedation if the patient is very anxious
- Furosemide (intravenously or intramuscularly)
- Consideration of whether to administer vasodilators ± positive inotropes
- Thoracocentesis and abdominocentesis as required.

Corneal ulcers – causes [12]

- Trauma/abrasions.
- Keratoconjunctivitis sicca.
- Foreign bodies.
- Infection (bacterial, viral, fungal).
- Exposure keratitis (e.g. due to an anatomical abnormality or nerve damage (facial nerve paralysis, trigeminal nerve paralysis)).
- Topical irritants.
- Entropion.
- Trichiasis.
- Distichiasis.
- Ectopic cilia.
- Dermoid.
- Eyelid agenesis.
- Eyelid neoplasia or inflammation.

NOTES

Cranial draw test [5]

Indications/Use

- To diagnose partial or complete rupture of the cranial cruciate ligament (CCL).
- NB This test does not identify isolated rupture of the caudolateral band of the CCL.
- Often used in association with the tibial compression test.

Contraindications

- Periarticular fibrosis and meniscal injury, with the caudal horn of the medial meniscus wedged between the femoral condyle and tibial plateau, may prevent cranial draw in a CCL-deficient stifle.

Patient preparation and positioning

- Can be performed in the conscious animal. However, if the patient is tense (due to pain or temperament) or if the CCL is only partially torn, sedation or general anaesthesia may be required.
- A conscious patient may be restrained in a standing position on three legs, with the affected limb held off the ground.
- Sedated or anaesthetized patients may be positioned in lateral recumbency, with the affected limb uppermost.

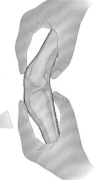

Technique

1. Grasp the distal femur in one hand, placing the thumb over the lateral fabella and the index finger on the patella.

   Cranial draw

2. Use the other hand to grasp the proximal tibia, placing the thumb over the head of the fibula and the index finger on the tibial crest.

3. Apply a cranial force to the tibia while the stifle joint is held in full extension, and then while the joint is held in 30–60 degrees of flexion.

Results

- Complete rupture of the CCL is associated with cranial displacement of the tibia relative to the femur, in both extension and flexion.
- Isolated rupture of the craniomedial band of the CCL is associated with cranial displacement of the tibia relative to the femur, in flexion only.
- A short cranial draw motion, with a distinct end point, may be detected in young animals and is normal.

NOTES

Cranial nerve tests [15]

Test	Afferent CN	Intermediate brain region	Efferent CN	Principal effect
Palpebral reflex	CN V – trigeminal (ophthalmic or maxillary)	Brainstem	CN VII – facial	Blink elicited by touching the medial or lateral canthus of the eye
Corneal sensation	CN V – trigeminal (ophthalmic)	Brainstem	CN VII – facial CN VI – abducent	Blink and globe retraction elicited by touching the cornea
Vestibulo-ocular reflex	CN VIII – vestibulocochlear	Brainstem	CN III – oculomotor CN IV – trochlear CN VI – abducent	Nystagmus induced by moving the head
Menace response	CN II – optic	Forebrain; cerebellum; brainstem	CN VII – facial	Blink elicited by a menacing gesture
Response to stimulation of nasal mucosa	CN V – trigeminal (ophthalmic)	Forebrain; brainstem	None	Withdrawal of the head elicited by touching the nasal mucosa
Pupillary light reflex	CN II – optic	Brainstem	CN III – oculomotor	Pupillary constriction elicited by shining a light in the eye
Gag reflex	CN IX – glossopharyngeal CN X – vagus	Brainstem	CN IX – glossopharyngeal CN X – vagus	Contraction of the pharynx elicited by its palpation

Cystocentesis [12]

Cystocentesis can be performed blind or with ultrasound guidance. Ultrasound guidance is preferred in animals where the bladder is not palpable, for example in small or obese patients.

- The patient should be firmly but gently restrained. It can be standing or in lateral or dorsal recumbency as preferred by the clinician.
- If a sterile sample is required, the patient should be clipped and the skin aseptically prepared over the region where the needle is to be introduced.
- A 21 or 23 G needle of appropriate length to pass through the body wall should be attached to a syringe.
- If ultrasound guidance is being used, the bladder should be identified. The needle should then be introduced into the bladder and the urine aspirated. The needle should be visible ultrasonographically. To achieve this, the needle should be kept in the same plane as the ultrasound probe and the needle introduced adjacent to the probe.
- If cystocentesis is being performed without ultrasound guidance, the bladder should be palpated and then pushed caudally and stabilized with the non-dominant hand.
- If the patient is in dorsal recumbency, the needle should be introduced between the caudal two mammary glands (midline in bitches and cats, and just lateral to the penis in male dogs).
- The needle should be directed into the bladder caudally at a 45-degree angle.
- Aspirate urine.
- Stop aspirating prior to removal of the needle.

NOTES

Decontamination [1, 27]

Dermal decontamination

Topical decontamination may be indicated for dermal exposure to a toxicant.

For detailed information see page 161 of the *BSAVA/VPIS Guide to Common Canine and Feline Poisons*.

Gastrointestinal decontamination

Decontamination consists of gastric evacuation (by emesis induction, gastric lavage or whole bowel irrigation) and administration of activated charcoal. However, there are several contraindications to gastric evacuation. These include:

- Ingestion of a caustic, corrosive, petroleum-based or volatile (resulting in aspiration pneumonia) substance
- Clinical signs of toxicosis (e.g. tremors, seizures, decreased level of consciousness, decreased gag reflex)
- Ingestion of the substance more than 2–3 hours prior to presentation (as it has now passed out of the stomach).

Induction of emesis

As gastric evacuation is time-dependent, animal poison control centres (e.g. the Veterinary Poisons Information Service) should be consulted to determine whether emesis induction is appropriate. If emesis is recommended, then this should be initiated at the earliest opportunity and generally within a maximum of 2–3 hours. Delayed induction of emesis (up to 4–6 hours following ingestion) is only recommended if the patient remains asymptomatic and if the toxicant is known to stay in the stomach for a prolonged period of time (e.g. chocolate, grapes, chewing gum containing xylitol).

Dogs: Apomorphine and hydrogen peroxide (3%) are equally effective emetic agents in dogs.

- Apomorphine – 0.03 mg/kg i.v. or 0.04 mg/kg i.m. is typically sufficient, although higher or repeated doses may be required. For subconjunctival administration, 6.25 mg tablets (typically) should be crushed. Side effects of apomorphine include sedation, bradycardia and protracted vomiting.

- Hydrogen peroxide (3%) – 1–5 ml/kg orally for up to two doses; maximum dose of 50 ml/dog. Side effects of hydrogen peroxide include protracted vomiting and haemorrhagic gastritis. Note: this product is not available in the UK.

Cats: Alpha-agonists (e.g. xylazine) are the only emetic agents recommended in cats. Apomorphine is typically ineffective in cats. Hydrogen peroxide is not generally recommended in cats due to the risk of severe haemorrhagic gastritis.

- Xylazine – 0.44 mg/kg i.m. Side effects include sedation and bradycardia, which can be reversed with yohimbine following emesis.

Sodium carbonate (washing soda) crystals are generally considered an effective emetic in both dogs and cats. The dose is empirical but typically a large crystal in a medium to large dog and a small crystal in a small dog or cat is sufficient. Caution is recommended as sodium carbonate is mildly caustic. The use of other emetics such as syrup of ipecac and household remedies (e.g. table salt, mustard) are no longer recommended due to the potentially severe side effects (e.g. severe haemorrhagic gastritis, intractable emesis, hypernatraemia).

It should be remembered that some emetics have a short delay before action. In addition, emetics have a prolonged duration of action (i.e. patients may continue to vomit for up to an hour following administration of an emetic agent). Thus, the use of an anti-emetic (e.g. maropitant) immediately following emesis may be beneficial.

Gastric lavage and whole bowel irrigation
See the *BSAVA Poisons database*.

Administration of activated charcoal

Activated charcoal is an absorbent. It must be administered as a powder or a slurry (rather than capsules or tablets) as its effectiveness is related to its surface area. Its large surface area binds toxicants through intermolecular and intra-molecular non-covalent bonds. Activated charcoal is available in many formulations (with and without an osmotic cathartic).

- Activated charcoal should only be administered when warranted and medically appropriate.
- When a toxicant cannot be identified but there is a high suspicion of poisoning, it is reasonable to give activated charcoal.

There are a number of toxicant- and patient-related contraindications to the administration of activated charcoal. These include:

Toxicant-related contraindications:

- Ingestion of corrosive or caustic agents
- Ingestion of hydrocarbons or petroleum distillates
- Ingestion of salt or other toxicants that can result in hypernatraemia
- Ingestion of toxicants known not to reliably bind to activated charcoal (e.g. heavy metals, ethylene glycol, xylitol).

Patient-related contraindications:

- Central nervous system depression
- Gastrointestinal disease (ileus, obstruction or perforation)
- Airway compromise or other condition predisposing to aspiration pneumonia
- Dehydration or hypovolaemia
- Electrolyte derangements or underlying disease where appropriate hydration and water balance is crucial (e.g. renal disease, diabetes mellitus)
- Endoscopy or surgery is imminent.

Dosage:

Activated charcoal should be administered as soon as possible following emesis or gastric lavage.

- Single dose – 1–5 g/kg (with an osmotic cathartic). ⟹

The use of an osmotic cathartic (e.g. sorbitol, magnesium sulphate) with the first dose is recommended to aid faecal expulsion.

Multiple doses of activated charcoal are warranted in the following situations:

- The toxicant undergoes enterohepatic circulation
- Ingestion of an extended-release drug
- Ingestion of drugs that have a long half-life
- Ingestion of a quantity of a drug approaching the LD50.

In these cases, the dosage of activated charcoal is as follows:

- Loading dose – 1–5 g/kg (with an osmotic cathartic)
  Repeat doses – 1–2 g/kg (without an osmotic cathartic) orally q6h for approximately 24 hours.

Ocular decontamination

See the *BSAVA Poisons database*.

Dehydration *see* Fluids – estimating percentage of dehydration

NOTES

Delmadinone [25, 26]
(Tardak) POM-V

Formulations: Injectable: 10 mg/ml suspension.

DOSES

Dogs: Benign prostatic hypertrophy 1.5–2 mg/kg (dogs <10 kg); 1–1.5 mg/kg (10–20 kg); 1 mg/kg (>20 kg) i.m., s.c. repeated after 8 days if no response. Animals that respond to treatment may need further treatment after 3–4 weeks.

Cats: Hypersexuality 1.5 mg/kg repeated after 8 days if no response. Animals that respond to treatment may need further treatment after 3–4 weeks.

Tardak 10 mg/ml Suspension (from datasheet)		
Patient bodyweight (kg)	Recommended dose (mg/kg)	Volume required (ml/kg)
Dogs and cats		
<10 kg	1.5–2.0	0.15–0.2
10–20 kg	1.0–1.5	0.10–0.15
>20 kg	1.0	0.10

Birds: 1 mg/kg i.m. once.

Mammals, Reptiles, Amphibians, Fish: No information available.

NOTES

Dental recording chart – cat [10]

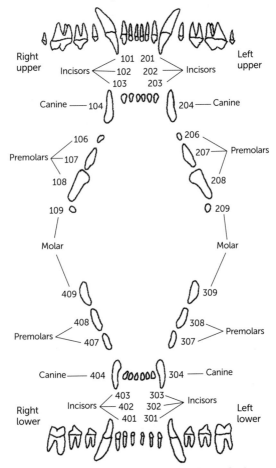

Right upper — Incisors ← 101 102 103 — 201 202 203 → Incisors — Left upper

Canine — 104 — 204 — Canine

Premolars ← 106 107 108 — 206 207 208 → Premolars

109 — 209

Molar — Molar

409 — 309

Premolars ← 408 407 — 308 307 → Premolars

Canine — 404 — 304 — Canine

Right lower — Incisors ← 403 402 401 — 303 302 301 → Incisors — Left lower

(Courtesy of Alexander M. Reiter, Dentistry and Oral Surgery Service, School of Veterinary Medicine, University of Pennsylvania)

Dental recording chart – dog [10]

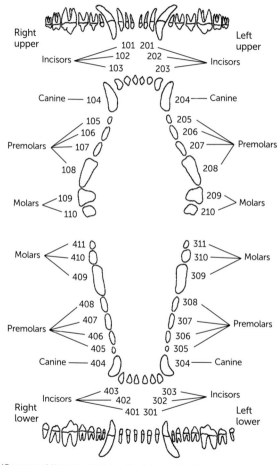

Right upper
Left upper

Incisors — 101 201 — Incisors
102 202
103 203

Canine — 104   204 — Canine

Premolars — 105   205 — Premolars
106   206
107   207
108
208

Molars — 109   209 — Molars
110   210

Molars — 411   311 — Molars
410   310
409   309

Premolars — 408   308 — Premolars
407   307
406   306
405   305

Canine — 404   304 — Canine

Incisors — 403 303 — Incisors
402 302
Right lower   401 301   Left lower

(Courtesy of Alexander M. Reiter, Dentistry and Oral Surgery Service, School of Veterinary Medicine, University of Pennsylvania)

Dexamethasone [25, 26]

(Aurizon, Dexadreson, Dexafort, Dexa-ject, Duphacort, Rapidexon, Voren, Dexamethasone*, Maxidex*, Maxitrol*) POM-V

Formulations:

- Ophthalmic: 0.1% solution (Maxidex, Maxitrol). Maxitrol also contains polymyxin B and neomycin.
- Injectable: 2 mg/ml solution; 1 mg/ml, 3 mg/ml suspension; 4 mg/ml (1.32 mg/ml sodium phosphate and 2.67 mg/ml of the phenylpropionate salts) (Voren); 2.5 mg/ml suspension with 7.5 mg/ml prednisolone.
- Topical: 0.9 mg/ml suspension with clotrimazole and marbofloxacin (Aurizon).
- Oral: 0.5 mg tablet. (1 mg of dexamethasone is equivalent to 1.1 mg of dexamethasone acetate, 1.3 mg of dexamethasone isonicotinate or dexamethasone sodium phosphate, or 1.4 mg of dexamethasone trioxa-undecanoate.)

DOSES

Dogs:

- Ophthalmic: Apply small amount of ointment to affected eye(s) q6–24h or 1 drop of solution in affected eye(s) q6–12h.
- Otic: 10 drops to ear once daily for 7–14 days (authorized dose; many authorities use less).
- Cerebral oedema: 2–3 mg/kg i.v., then 1 mg/kg s.c. q6–8h, taper off.
- Hypoadrenocorticism: 0.2 mg/kg i.v. repeat daily until able to use oral medication.
- Inflammation: 0.01–0.16 mg/kg i.m., s.c., p.o. q24h for 3–5 days maximum.
- Prevention and treatment of anaphylaxis: 0.5 mg/kg i.v. once.
- Immunosuppression: 0.3–0.64 mg/kg i.m., s.c., p.o. q24h for up to 5 days.
- Assessment of adrenal function: low dose dexamethasone suppression test (0.015 mg/kg i.v.).

Cats:

- Ophthalmic, Cerebral oedema, Inflammation, Anaphylaxis, Immunosuppression: doses as for dogs.
- Assessment of adrenal function: dexamethasone suppression test (0.15 mg/kg i.v.). Note difference to dogs.

Mammals: Ophthalmic: Apply small amount of ointment to affected eye(s) q6–24h or 1 drop of solution in affected eye(s) q6–12h.

- Primates: 0.5–2 mg/kg i.v., i.m., s.c. once (cerebral oedema); 0.25–1 mg/kg i.v., i.m., s.c. q24h (inflammation)
- Ferrets: 0.5–2.0 mg/kg s.c., i.m., i.v. q24h; 1 mg/kg i.m., i.v. once followed with prednisolone (post adrenalectomy)
- Rabbits: 0.2–0.6 mg/kg s.c., i.m., i.v. q24h
- Guinea pigs: 0.6 mg/kg i.v., i.m., s.c. q24h (pregnancy toxaemia)
- Others: anti-inflammatory: 0.055–0.2 mg/kg i.m., s.c. q12–24h tapering dose over 3–14 days.

Birds: 2–6 mg/kg i.v., i.m. q12–24h.

Reptiles: Inflammatory, non-infectious respiratory disease: 2–4 mg/kg i.m., i.v. q24h for 3 days.

Amphibians: 1.5 mg/kg s.c., i.m. q24h.

Fish: 1–2 mg/kg i.m., intraperitoneal or 10 mg/l for 60 minute bath q12–24h.

NOTES

Dexmedetomidine [25, 26]
(Dexdomitor, Sileo) POM-V

Formulations:

- Injectable: 0.1 mg/ml, 0.5 mg/ml solution.
- Oral: 0.1 mg/ml gel.

DOSES

Dogs: Control of noise related anxiety 125 µg (micrograms)/m^2 applied to the oral mucosa as a gel 30–60 minutes before the onset of the noise stimulus, or after the first signs. Dosing can be repeated after 2–3 hours for a maximum of occasions.

Dogs, Cats:

- Premedication: 3–10 µg (micrograms)/kg i.v., i.m, s.c. in combination with an opioid (use lower end of dose range i.v.).
- Emergence excitation: 1 µg (microgram)/kg i.v. can be given to manage emergence excitation during recovery from anaesthesia, although administration around the time of extubation will prolong the recovery period from anaesthesia and treated animals should be monitored carefully.
- Perioperative analgesia and rousable sedation: 1–2 µg (micrograms)/kg/h constant rate infusion is indicated, although the efficacy of analgesia will be improved in most animals if dexmedetomidine is used as an adjunct to opioid analgesia.

Mammals:

- Ferrets 0.04–0.1 mg/kg s.c., i.m.
- Rabbits: 0.025–0.05 mg/kg i.v. or 0.05–0.15 mg/kg s.c., i.m.

Birds:

- Buzzards: 0.1 mg atropine + 25 µg (micrograms)/kg dexmedetomidine i.m.
- Kestrels: 0.05 mg atropine + 75 µg (micrograms)/kg dexmedetomidine i.m. as induction for isoflurane general anaesthesia. Reversed when bird is stable with 250 µg atipamezole i.m.

Reptiles: Usually combined with ketamine and/or opioids/midazolam to provide light anaesthesia.

Amphibians, Fish: No information available.

See also Sedation combinations

NOTES

Diazepam [25, 26]

(Diazemuls*, Diazepam Rectubes*, Stesolid*, Valium* and several others) POM

Formulations:

- Injectable: 5 mg/ml emulsion (2 ml ampoules, Diazemuls).
- Oral: 2 mg, 5 mg, 10 mg tablets; 2 mg/5 ml solution.
- Rectal: 2 mg/ml (1.25, 2.5 ml tubes), 4 mg/ml (2.5 ml tubes) solutions; 10 mg suppositories.

DOSES

Dogs:

- Anxiolytic: 0.5–2.0 mg/kg p.o as required.
- Sedation and premedication: 0.2–0.5 mg/kg i.v., i.m.
- Skeletal muscle relaxation: 2–10 mg/dog p.o. q8–12h.
- Emergency management of seizures, including status epilepticus: bolus dose of 0.5–1 mg/kg i.v. or intrarectally (if venous access is not available). Time to onset of clinical effect is 2–3 min for i.v. use; therefore, repeat every 10 min if no clinical effect, up to three times. Additional doses may be administered if appropriate supportive care facilities are available (for support of respiration). Constant rate i.v. infusion for control of status epilepticus or cluster seizures: initial rate 0.5–2 mg/kg/h, titrated to effect.

Cats:

- Anxiolytic: 0.2–0.4 mg/kg p.o. q8h.
- Appetite stimulant: 0.1–0.2 mg/kg i.v. once.
- Behavioural modification of urine spraying and muscle relaxation: 1.25–5 mg/cat p.o. q8h. The dose should be gradually increased to achieve the desired effect without concurrent sedation.
- Emergency management of seizures including status epilepticus: bolus dose of 0.5–1 mg/kg i.v. or intrarectally if venous access is not available. Time to onset of clinical effect is 2–3 min for i.v. use, therefore, repeat every 10 min if there is no clinical effect, up to maximum

of three times. Constant rate i.v. infusion for the control of status epilepticus or cluster seizures: initial rate of 0.5 mg/kg/h. Care should be taken in cats to avoid overdosing: if cats demonstrate excessive sedation then diazepam should be discontinued. Consider monitoring liver parameters.

Mammals:
- Primates: sedation and seizures: 0.5–1 mg/kg p.o., i.m.
- Sugar gliders, Hedgehogs: sedation and seizures: 0.5–2 mg/kg p.o., s.c., i.m.
- Ferrets: seizures: 2–5 mg/kg i.m. once; urethral sphincter muscle relaxation post urinary catheterization or obstruction: 0.5 mg/kg p.o., i.m., i.v. q6–8h
- Rabbits: epileptic seizures, pre-anaesthetic sedation, muscle relaxation: 1–5 mg/kg i.v.
- Guinea pigs: 0.5–5.0 mg/kg i.m. as required
- Chinchillas, Hamsters, Gerbils, Rats, Mice: 2.5–5 mg/kg i.m., intraperitoneal once.

Birds: Epileptic seizures: 0.1–1 mg/kg i.v., i.m. once
- Raptors: Appetite stimulant: 0.2 mg/kg p.o. q24h.

Reptiles: Epileptic seizures: 2.5 mg/kg i.m., i.v.

Amphibians, Fish: No information available.

See also Sedation combinations

NOTES

Doxycycline [25, 26]

(Doxyseptin 300, Ornicure, Pulmodox, Ronaxan, Vibramycin*, Vibravenos*) POM-V

Formulations:

- Oral: 20 mg, 100 mg tablets (Ronaxan), 300 mg tablets (Doxyseptin); 260 mg/sachet powder (Ornicure).
- Injectable: 20 mg/ml long-acting injection (Vibravenos; import on an STC).

DOSES

Dogs, Cats: 10 mg/kg p.o. q24h with food.

Mammals:

- Primates: 3–4 mg/kg p.o. q12h
- Hedgehogs: 2.5–10 mg/kg p.o., s.c., i.m. q12h
- Rabbits: 2.5–4 mg/kg p.o. q24h
- Rats, Mice: 5 mg/kg p.o. q12h
- Other rodents: 2.5 mg/kg p.o. q12h or 70–100 mg/kg s.c., i.m. of the long-acting preparation (Vibravenos); however, this is not currently permitted under the STA required to import this product.

Birds:

- Raptors: 50 mg/kg p.o. q12h, 100 mg/kg i.m. q7d (Vibravenos)
- Parrots: 15–50 mg/kg p.o. q24h, 1000 mg/kg in soft food/dehulled seed, 75–100 mg/kg i.m. q7d (Vibravenos; lowest dose rate for macaws); course of treatment with doxycycline for chlamydophilosis = 45 days
- Passerines/Pigeons: 40 mg/kg p.o. 12–24h, 200–500 mg/l in water (soft or deionized water only).

Reptiles: 50 mg/kg i.m. once, then 25 mg/kg i.m. q72h.

Amphibians: 50 mg/kg i.m. q7d.

Fish: No information available.

Drug distribution categories [25, 26]

Authorized small animal medicines within Great Britain now fall within the first four categories below and all packaging supplied by drug manufacturers and distributors was changed in 2008. Medical products not authorized for veterinary use retain their former classification (e.g. GSL, P, POM). Other laws apply in other jurisdictions. Some nutritional supplements (nutraceuticals) are not considered medicinal products and therefore are not classified. Where a product does not have a marketing authorization it is designated 'general sale'.

AVM-GSL: Authorized veterinary medicine – general sales list. This may be sold by anyone.

NFA-VPS: Non-food animal medicine – veterinarian, pharmacist, Suitably Qualified Person (SQP). These medicines for companion animals must be supplied by a veterinary surgeon, pharmacist or SQP. An SQP has to be registered with the Animal Medicines Training Regulatory Authority (AMTRA). Veterinary nurses can become SQPs but it is not automatic.

POM-VPS: Prescription-only medicine – veterinarian, pharmacist, SQP (formerly PML livestock products, MFSX products and a few P products). These medicines for food-producing animals (including horses) can only be supplied on an oral or written veterinary prescription from a veterinary surgeon, pharmacist or SQP and can only be supplied by one of those groups of people in accordance with the prescription.

POM-V: Prescription-only medicine – veterinarian. These medicines can only be supplied against a veterinary prescription that has been prepared (either orally or in writing) by a veterinary surgeon to animals under their care following a clinical assessment, and can only be supplied by a veterinary surgeon or pharmacist in accordance with the prescription.

Exemptions for Small Pet Animals (ESPA): Schedule 6 of the Veterinary Medicine Regulations 2013 (unofficially known as the Small Animal Exemption Scheme) allows for the use of medicines in certain pet species (aquarium fish, cage birds, ferrets, homing pigeons, rabbits, small rodents and terrarium animals) the active ingredient of which has been declared by the Secretary of State as not requiring veterinary control. These medicines are exempt from the requirement for a marketing authorization and are not therefore required to prove safety, quality or efficacy, but must be manufactured to the same standards as authorized medicines and are subject to pharmacovigilance reporting.

CD: Controlled Drug. A substance controlled by the Misuse of Drugs Act 1971 and Regulations. The CD is followed by (Schedule 1), (Schedule 2), (Schedule 3), (Schedule 4) or (Schedule 5) depending on the Schedule to The Misuse of Drugs Regulations 2001 (as amended) in which the preparation is included. You could be prosecuted for failure to comply with this act. Prescribers are reminded that there are additional requirements relating to the prescribing of Controlled Drugs. For more information see the *BSAVA Guide to the Use of Veterinary Medicines* at www.bsava.com.

Schedule 1: Includes LSD, cannabis, lysergide and other drugs that are not used medicinally. Possession and supply are prohibited except in accordance with Home Office Authority.

Schedule 2: Includes etorphine, ketamine, morphine, methadone, pethidine, secobarbital (quinalbarbitone), diamorphine (heroin), cocaine and amphetamine. Record all purchases and each individual supply (within 24 hours). Registers must be kept for 2 calendar years after the last entry. Drugs must be kept under safe custody (locked secure cabinet), except secobarbital. There are specific requirements regarding the destruction of Schedule 2 Controlled Drugs, which may require an independent veterinary surgeon or person authorized by the Secretary of State to witness.

Schedule 3: Includes buprenorphine, tramadol, the barbiturates (e.g. pentobarbital and phenobarbital but not secobarbital – which is Schedule 2), midazolam and others. Buprenorphine, with some others, must be kept under safe custody (locked secure cabinet) and it is advisable that all Schedule 3 drugs are locked away (although not compulsory for the rest). Retention of invoices for 2 years is necessary.

Schedule 4: Includes most of the benzodiazepines except midazolam (which is Schedule 3), and androgenic and anabolic steroids (e.g. nandralone). Exempted from control when used in normal veterinary practice.

Schedule 5: Includes preparations (such as several codeine products) which, because of their strength, are exempt from virtually all Controlled Drug requirements other than the retention of invoices for 2 years.

NOTES

Dystocia — general approach [12, 17]

Diagnosis

Clinical signs

Within the clinical history the following criteria are useful in indicating the likely presence of dystocia:

- There has been a reduction in rectal temperature (which may have returned to normal, be above normal or remained low) commencing more than 12 hours previously and there are no signs of parturition
- There has been passage of a green (bitch) or red–brown (queen) discharge from the vulva, which originates from the marginal haematoma and indicates that at least one placenta is beginning to become separated
- There has been expulsion of fetal fluids, commencing 2–4 hours previously, and no progression of parturition
- There has been cessation of signs of parturition for more than 2 hours, or infrequent signs of parturition for more than 2–4 hours
- There have been strong signs of parturition for more than 30 minutes but no signs of fetal expulsion
- There is other evidence of probable dystocia (e.g. a fetus is visibly stuck in the birth canal)
- The dam is depressed, lethargic or showing signs of shock, fluid loss or dehydration.

Non-obstructive dystocia: In females with non-obstructive dystocia the common presentation is with relaxation of the perineal musculature, dilatation of the cervix (this can only be assessed upon endoscopic examination and not digital palpation) and having already had a decline in plasma progesterone (and in bitches a subsequent decline in rectal temperature). When placental separation occurs, a green (bitch) or red–brown (queen) vulval discharge will be evident. Early in the course of the condition the fetuses will be alive, fetal movement may be palpated, and fetal movement and heartbeats may be detected ultrasonographically. Fetal death can be recognized immediately using ultrasonography by an absence of fetal movement and by a non-moving echogenic appearance to the heart. When these animals are presented later, fetal death can be detected radiographically by a change in the fetal posture, by the accumulation of gas within the fetus and/or uterus, and by the overlapping of the bones of the fetal skull, although these changes may take several days before they are evident.

Obstructive dystocia: In females with obstructive dystocia, whilst there may be similar confirmatory signs, there is usually a history of active parturition with significant straining that has been non-productive. Usually fetuses can be identified lodged within the birth canal as a result of fetal or maternal abnormalities.

Key indications for veterinary intervention

Indications for veterinary intervention

- Abnormal vaginal/vulval discharge
- No onset of Stage 2 labour (primary uterine inertia)
- Stage 2 labour >4 hours without fetal delivery
- >2 hours between fetal deliveries
- >30 minutes active straining without fetal delivery
- >1 hour weak intermittent straining without fetal delivery
- Evidence of maternal distress
- Evidence of fetal distress (heart rate <180 bpm or <2 x maternal heart rate)

Indications for surgical intervention

- No onset of Stage 2 labour (primary uterine inertia)
- Non-obstructive uterine inertia refractory to medical treatment
- Feto-maternal disproportion
- Systemic maternal illness
- Evidence of maternal distress refractory to medical treatment
- Evidence of marked fetal distress (heart rate <150 bpm)
- Prolonged Stage 2 labour with multiple fetuses in absence of obstruction

NOTES

Dystocia in queens [22]

Dystocia may be diagnosed in queens when:

- Normal delivery is interrupted (obstruction or secondary uterine inertia):
  - A kitten and/or membranes are visible at the vulva for over 15 minutes with no progress
  - >3 hours have passed between delivery of individual kittens
  - No kittens have been produced after 3–4 hours of Stage 2 labour
  - Strong contractions are present for >60 minutes with no kitten delivered
  - Failure to deliver all kittens within 36 hours (the vast majority of normal parturitions are complete by 24 hours, although very rarely normal parturition can take up to 42 hours)
- Normal labour is not initiated at term (primary inertia)
  - queen is >1 week overdue
- Maternal health is compromised:
  - Queen is distressed and biting at the vulvar area
  - Serious systemic illness in the queen
  - Abnormal vulvar discharge (e.g. profuse haemorrhage, green discharge with foul odour)
- Fetal distress is diagnosed (heart rate <150–160 beats/min; normal fetal heart rate is 193–263 beats/min).

Accurate diagnosis of the cause of dystocia is necessary to determine whether medical or surgical intervention is most appropriate.

The diagnostic plan for dystocia in queens should include:

- Collection of a reproductive and medical history (current health status, concurrent diseases, drugs or supplements being administered, details of previous pregnancies, etc.)
- Physical examination (including abdominal palpation for uterine size and position, palpation of the pelvis via the rectum to detect obstruction, vaginal examination for the presence of a kitten)

- Laboratory testing (minimum data required: haematology, serum calcium and glucose to determine if supplementation is necessary)
- Abdominal radiographs (evaluate fetal size, number and position)
- Evaluation of fetal condition with ultrasonography (fetal movement, fetal heart rates) or Doppler probe applied to the abdomen (heart rates only), when available.

NOTES

Ear disease – topical polypharmaceuticals [25, 26]

The following POM-V preparations contain two or more drugs and are used topically in the ear. There are a number of AVM-GSL preparations used for ear cleaning etc. that are not listed here.

Trade name	Antibacterial	Steroid	Antifungal
Aurizon	Marbofloxacin	Dexamethasone	Clotrimazole
Canaural[a]	Fusidic acid Framycetin	Prednisolone	Nystatin
Easotic	Gentamicin	Hydrocortisone aceponate	Miconazole
Osurnia	Florphenicol	Betamethasone	Terbinafine
Otomax	Gentamicin	Betamethasone	Clotrimazole
Posatex	Orbifloxacin	Mometasone	Posaconozole
Surolan[a]	Polymixin B	Prednisolone	Miconazole

[a]Note that there is some evidence from clinical trials that products that do not contain a specific acaricidal compound may nevertheless be effective at treating infestations of ear mites. The mode of action is unclear but the vehicle for these polypharmaceutical products may be involved.

NOTES

ECG standard leads, lead II diagram and reference ranges [5]

Standard leads for electrocardiography

Lead	Attachment site	Colour
RA ('right arm')	Right elbow	Red
LA ('left arm')	Left elbow	Yellow
F or LL ('left leg')	Left stifle	Green
N or RL ('right leg', earth lead)	Right stifle	Black

Lead II at 1 cm/mV and 50 mm/s

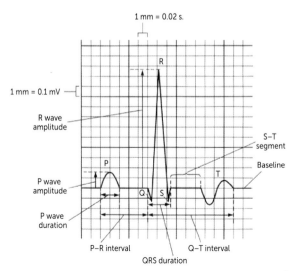

Reference ranges

Parameter	Unit	Dogs	Cats
Heart rate	Beats per minute	70–160 for adult dogs	120–240
		60–140 for giant breeds	
		Up to 180 for toy breeds	
		Up to 220 for puppies	
P wave duration	Seconds	<0.04 (<0.05 in giant breeds)	<0.04
P wave amplitude	mV	<0.4	<0.2
P–R interval	Seconds	0.06–0.13	0.05–0.09
QRS duration	Seconds	<0.06	<0.04
R wave amplitude	mV	<2.5–3.0	<0.9
Q–T interval	Seconds	0.15–0.25	0.12–0.18
Mean electrical axis (MEA)	Degrees	+40 to +100	0 to +160

Data from Tilley LP (1992) *Essentials of Canine and Feline Electrocardiography: Interpretation and Management, 3rd edn.* Philadelphia, Lea & Febiger.

Emesis induction *see* Decontamination

NOTES

Endotracheal tube sizes [6]

Sizes (internal diameter) (mm)	Cuffed and/or uncuffed	Approximate lean bodyweight (kg)
2.0, 2.5, 3.0	Cuffed and uncuffed	1–2.5
3.5, 4.0, 4.5	Cuffed and uncuffed	2.5–5
5, 6	Cuffed and uncuffed (size 5)	4–9
7, 8	Cuffed	7–15
9, 10	Cuffed	15–25
11, 12	Cuffed	25–45
14, 16	Cuffed	>40

Suggested sizes of endotracheal tubes suitable for small animal practice. Note that there is large individual variation in tracheal diameter in dogs and this table is intended as a guideline only. Brachycephalic breeds may have a hypoplastic (narrow) trachea.

Enrofloxacin [25, 26]

(Baytril, Enrocare, Enrotab, Enrotron, Enrox, Enroxil, Fenoflox, Floxabactin, Floxibac, Powerflox, Quinoflox, Xeden, Zobuxa) POM-V

Formulations:
- Injectable: 25 mg/ml, 50 mg/ml, 100 mg/ml solutions.
- Oral: 15 mg, 50 mg, 100 mg, 150 mg, 200 mg, 250 mg tablets; 25 mg/ml solution.

DOSES

Dogs, Cats: 5 mg/kg s.c. q24h; 2.5 mg/kg p.o. q12h or 5 mg/kg p.o. q24h. Some isolates of *Pseudomonas aeruginosa* may require higher doses, contact the manufacturer to discuss individual cases.

⟩⟩⟩

Baytril Flavour Tablets (from datasheet)				
Dose rate	No. of tablets per total daily dose			
	15 mg	*50 mg*	*150 mg*	*250 mg*
Cats and small dogs				
5 mg/kg once daily or as a divided dose twice daily for 3 to 10 days	1 per 3 kg bodyweight			
Medium dogs				
5 mg/kg once daily or as a divided dose twice daily for 3 to 10 days		1 per 10 kg bodyweight		
Large dogs				
5 mg/kg once daily or as a divided dose twice daily for 3 to 10 days			1 per 30 kg bodyweight	1 per 50 kg bodyweight

Mammals:
- Ferrets: 5–10 mg/kg p.o., s.c., i.m. q12h or 10–20 mg/kg p.o., s.c., i.m. q24h
- Rabbits: 10–20 mg/kg p.o., s.c., i.v. q24h
- Rodents: 5–20 mg/kg s.c., p.o. q12–24h
- Others: 5–10 mg/kg s.c., p.o. q12h or 20 mg/kg s.c., p.o. q24h.

Birds: 10 mg/kg p.o., i.m. q12h (licensed dose) or 100–200 mg/l drinking water.

Reptiles: Variable absorption when given p.o. so i.m. administration may be more appropriate in critically ill animals. Most species: 5–10 mg/kg i.m., p.o. q24–48h

- Indian star tortoises: 5 mg/kg i.m. q12–24h
- Gopher tortoises: 5 mg/kg i.m. q24–48h

- Red-eared sliders: 5 mg/kg i.m. or 10 mg/kg p.o., i.m., s.c., intracoelomic q24h or 500 mg/l as a 6–8 h bath q24h
- Savannah monitors: 10 mg/kg i.m. q5d
- Green iguanas: 5 mg/kg p.o., i.m. q24h
- Burmese pythons: 10 mg/kg i.m., then q48h
- Pit vipers: 10 mg/kg i.m. q48–72h.

Amphibians: 5–10 mg/kg p.o., s.c., i.m. q24h.

Fish: 5–10 mg/kg i.m., intraperitoneal, p.o. q24–48h for 7 doses or 2.5–5 mg/l by immersion for 5 h q24–48h for 5–7 treatments.

Ethylene glycol poisoning (URGENT) [1]
Also known as: ethanediol, antifreeze

Description/exposure

Ethylene glycol is a clear, odourless compound commonly found in high concentrations in radiator fluid, antifreeze, de-icing solutions and some industrial solvents. It is also found in low concentrations in paints, ink jet printers and caulking material, but these rarely result in toxicosis.

Mechanism of action

Ethylene glycol itself is not poisonous; rather it is the metabolites of ethylene glycol that result in severe toxicosis. Hence, the goal of antidotal therapy for ethylene glycol toxicosis is to prevent the metabolism of ethylene glycol to these dangerous metabolites. Metabolism occurs primarily in the liver where alcohol dehydrogenase converts ethylene glycol to glycoaldehyde, glycolic acid, glyoxylic acid and oxalic acid. These metabolites can cause cardio-pulmonary failure, metabolic acidosis, central nervous system (CNS) depression and kidney injury. Oxalic acid can precipitate to crystals of calcium oxalate monohydrate in the tubular lumen of the kidneys, resulting in secondary acute kidney injury (AKI).

⟩⟩⟩

Clinical presentation

CNS signs (e.g. ataxia, depression), profound polyuria/
polydipsia and gastrointestinal signs (e.g. hypersalivation,
vomiting) may be seen as soon as 30 minutes after
ingestion. CNS depression typically resolves within 12 hours
in dogs. Clinical signs of AKI (e.g. gastrointestinal signs,
ptyalism, uraemic halitosis, oral ulceration, depression,
anorexia, abdominal pain, oliguria, anuria) typically do
not develop until 24–72 hours following exposure. Once
azotaemia has developed, the prognosis is grave,
despite treatment.

Diagnostics

A range of tests can be used to help diagnose ethylene
glycol toxicosis, although numerous false-positive results
can be seen with propylene glycol (found in diazepam,
methocarbamol and other injectable agents), activated
charcoal containing sorbitol, isopropyl alcohol and ethanol.
Rapid quantitative measurement of blood levels is the most
accurate way of diagnosing ethylene glycol toxicosis, but
this is not commonly available. Other clinicopathological
changes seen with ethylene glycol toxicosis include
metabolic acidosis (identified by a high anion gap and low
bicarbonate level) with normochloraemia. This can develop
quite rapidly and can be severe. Ionized hypocalcaemia and
hyperglycaemia are also very common, occurring in >50%
of dogs and cats. Calcium oxalate crystalluria can be seen
3–8 hours post-exposure. In addition, the osmolar gap can
be calculated and compared with the measured osmolar
gap. The presence of a high osmolar gap is consistent with
ethylene glycol toxicosis, but can also be seen with lactic
acidosis and uraemia. Hyperphosphataemia and azotaemia
are appreciated as AKI develops.

Treatment

Ethylene glycol is rapidly absorbed from the gastrointestinal
tract, thus performing gastrointestinal decontamination
more than 1 hour after exposure is not indicated.

Activated charcoal does not reliably bind to ethylene glycol and is not typically warranted. Therapy should be targeted at preventing the metabolism of ethylene glycol to its metabolites. Ethanol or fomepizole/4-methylpyrazole (4-MP) can be used as both have a stronger affinity for alcohol dehydrogenase than ethylene glycol. Antidotal therapy must be initiated within 3 hours of exposure in cats, and within 8-12 hours in dogs, for the best outcome. In cats, antidotal treatment initiated more than 3 hours following exposure is ineffective and these cases are associated with an almost 100% fatality rate.

- Fomepizole
  - Cats: 125 mg/kg i.v. initially followed by 31.25 mg/kg i.v. at 12, 24 and 36 hours post-exposure
  - Dogs: 20 mg/kg i.v. initially followed by 15 mg/kg i.v. at 12 and 24 hours post-exposure, and then 5 mg/kg i.v. at 36 hours post-exposure

Side effects of antidotal therapy can be seen but are typically mild. Ethanol is associated with CNS depression and may further contribute to the metabolic acidosis (through the conversion of pyruvate to lactate) and hypoglycaemia. These side effects are generally not seen with 4-MP, which is generally considered to be safer. However, 4-MP is expensive and not always available. The use of haemodialysis (if available) can be considered both to remove ethylene glycol (and its metabolites) prior to the onset of clinical signs and to treat AKI.

Prognosis

Cats treated within 3 hours and dogs treated within 8–12 hours with 4-MP or ethanol have a fair prognosis. The presence of azotaemia or the progression to anuric AKI represents a grave prognosis.

NOTES

FAST scan – abdominal [20]

Positioning and preparation

- Right lateral recumbency is recommended, as this is also the best position for abdominocentesis, electrocardiography and echocardiography. However, this procedure can be carried out in a standing animal.
- One of the benefits of this procedure is that it can often be carried out in the conscious patient.

Technique

Placing the ultrasound probe on the four areas shown and scanning widely in both sagittal and transverse planes gives the best chance of detecting more subtle fluid accumulation (see below).

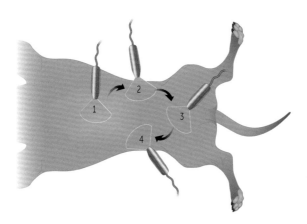

Four-point ultrasound assessment for free abdominal fluid.
1 = diaphragmaticohepatic; 2 = splenorenal; 3 = cystocolic;
4 = hepatorenal. (Redrawn after Lisciandro et al., 2009)

⟾

Limitations

- There is always the possibility of false-positive or false-negative results. For example, the gall bladder and common bile duct can appear as hypoechoic sharp angles, similar to free fluid, depending on the plane of imaging.
- If in doubt, the scan should be repeated on a regular basis to detect any changes.

Febantel *see* Pyrantel

NOTES

Fenbendazole [25, 26]

(Bob Martin Easy to Use Wormer, Granofen, Lapizole, Panacur, Various authorized proprietary products, Zerofen) AVM-GSL, NFA-VPS

Formulations: Oral: 222 mg/g granules (22%); 20 mg/ml oral suspension (2%); 25 mg/ml oral suspension (2.5%); 100 mg/ml oral suspension (10%); 187.5 mg/g oral paste (18.75%).

DOSES

Dogs:
- Roundworms, tapeworms: dogs <6 months old: 50 mg/kg p.o. q24h for 3 consecutive days; >6 months old: 100 mg/kg as a single dose p.o. Treatment of *Capillaria* may need to be extended to 10 days. Repeat q3months. For pregnant bitches 25 mg/kg p.o. q24h from day 40 until 2 days post-whelping (approximately 25 days)
- *Angiostrongylus vasorum*: 50 mg/kg p.o. for a minimum of 10 days, although the duration of treatment has yet to be defined
- *Oslerus osleri*: 50 mg/kg p.o. q24h for 7 days, although a repeat course of treatment may be required in some cases
- *Aelurostrongylus abstrusus*: 20 mg/kg p.o. q24h for 3 days
- Giardiasis: 50 mg/kg p.o. q24h for 5 days.

Cats:
- Roundworms, tapeworms: cats <6 months old: 20 mg/kg p.o. q24h for 5 days; >6 months old: 100 mg/kg as a single dose p.o.
- *Aelurostrongylus abstrusus*: 20 mg/kg p.o. q24h for 5 days
- Giardiasis: 20 mg/kg p.o. for 5 days.

Panacur (from datasheet)

Dose rate	Patient bodyweight	Volume required
2.5% ORAL SUSPENSION		
Adult dogs and cats		
100 mg/kg or 4 ml/kg	250 g	1 ml
	500 g	2 ml
	750 g	3 ml
	1 kg	4 ml
	1.5 kg	6 ml
	2 kg	8 ml
	2.5 kg	10 ml
Puppies and kittens under 6 months of age		
50 mg/kg or 2 ml/kg daily for 3 consecutive days	250 g	0.5 ml daily for 3 days
	500 g	1 ml daily for 3 days
	1 kg	2 ml daily for 3 days
	1.5 kg	3 ml daily for 3 days
	2 kg	4 ml daily for 3 days
Pregnant dogs		
25 mg/kg or 1 ml/kg (from day 40 of pregnancy continuously to 2 days post-whelping)	2–4 kg	4 ml daily for approximately 25 days
	4–8 kg	8 ml daily for approximately 25 days
	8–16 kg	16 ml daily for approximately 25 days
10% ORAL SUSPENSION		
Adult dogs and cats		
100 mg/kg or 1 ml/kg	2–4 kg	4 ml
	4–8 kg	8 ml
	8–16 kg	16 ml
	16–24 kg	24 ml
	24–32 kg	32 ml
	32–64 kg	64 ml

Panacur (from datasheet)		
Dose rate	Patient bodyweight	Volume required
Puppies and kittens under 6 months of age		
50 mg/kg or 0.5 ml/kg daily for 3 consecutive days	<1 kg	0.5 ml daily for 3 days
	1–2 kg	1 ml daily for 3 days
	2–4 kg	2 ml daily for 3 days
	4–6 kg	3 ml daily for 3 days
	6–8 kg	4 ml daily for 3 days
	8–10 kg	5 ml daily for 3 days
Pregnant dogs		
25 mg/kg or 1 ml/4 kg (from day 40 of pregnancy continuously to 2 days post-whelping)	4 kg	1 ml daily for approximately 25 days
	8 kg	2 ml daily for approximately 25 days
	12 kg	3 ml daily for approximately 25 days
	20 kg	5 ml daily for approximately 25 days
	40 kg	10 ml daily for approximately 25 days

Mammals:

- Primates: 50 mg/kg p.o. q24h for 3 days
- Sugar gliders: 20–50 mg/kg p.o. q24h for 3 days, repeat in 14 days
- Hedgehogs: 25 mg/kg p.o., repeat at 14 and 28 days
- Rabbits: E. cuniculi: 20 mg/kg p.o. q24h for 28 days; Oxyuriasis: 50ppm (50 mg/kg) in feed for 5 days
- Other small mammals: 20–50 mg/kg p.o. q24h for 5 consecutive days; the higher end of the range is suggested for giardiasis only.

Birds:

- Nematodes: 20–100 mg/kg p.o., administer 2 doses separated by 10 days; capillariasis: 25 mg/kg p.o. q24h for 5 consecutive days; Pigeons: 16 mg/kg p.o. once, repeat after 10 days if necessary or 10–20 mg/kg p.o. ⟩⟩⟩

q24h for 3 days, repeat after 2 weeks; Passerines:
20 mg/kg p.o. q24h for 3 doses. Not advisable to give
more than 50 mg/kg in unfamiliar species.
- Giardiasis: 50 mg/kg p.o. q24h for 3 doses.

Reptiles:
- Nematodes: 50–100 mg/kg p.o., per cloaca once or
  20–25 mg/kg p.o., per cloaca q24h over 3–5 day
  course. Repeated doses have been advised but may be
  unnecessary as complete effect may not be seen until
  31 days post-treatment.
- Giardiasis and flagellates: 50 mg/kg p.o. q24h for 3–5
  days.

Amphibians: 100 mg/kg p.o., repeat in 2 weeks.

Fish: External monogenean parasites: 25 mg/l by immersion
for 12 h; Gastrointestinal nematodes: 50 mg/kg p.o. q24h for
2 days, repeat in 14 days.

NOTES

Ferret biological data [21]

Lifespan (years)	8–10 (max. 15); 5–7 in the USA
Average bodyweight (g)	Males: 1200 Females: 600
Rectal temperature (°C)	38.8 (37.8–40)
Heart rate (beats/min)	200–250
Respiration rate (breaths/min)	33–36

Fipronil [25, 26]

(Broadline, Certifect, Effipro, Eliminall, Felevox, Fiprospot, Frontline, Frontect and many others) AVM-GSL, NFA-VPS, POM-V

Formulations: Topical: 10% w/v fipronil spot-on pipettes in a wide range of sizes, (Frontline and many others); some formulations combined with other drugs including; S-methoprene (Frontline Combo/Plus); permethrin (Frontect) amitraz, eprinomectin and praziquantel (Certifect). Also 0.25% w/v fipronil spray in alcohol base (Effipro and Frontline sprays) in a range of sizes.

DOSES

Dogs:
- Flea infestations: spray 3–6 ml/kg (6–12 pumps/kg 100 ml application, 2–4 pumps/kg 250 ml or 500 ml application) or apply 1 pipette per dog according to bodyweight. Treatment should be repeated not more frequently than every 4 weeks.
- *Neotrombicula autumnalis*, *Sarcoptes* spp. and *Cheyletiella* spp. infestations: spray should be used every 1–2 weeks.

Cats: Spray 3–6 ml/kg (6–12 pumps/kg 100 ml application) or apply 1 pipette per cat. Treatment should be repeated monthly.

⟩

Mammals:
- Ferrets: spray 3–6 ml/kg (6–12 pumps/kg 100 ml application) q30–60d
- Rodents: 7.5 mg/kg topically (15 pumps/kg 100 ml application) q30–60d
- Other mammals: apply lightly q14d. Do not use in rabbits.

Birds: Use spray form q30–60d. Apply to cotton wool and dab behind head, under wings and at base of tail (raptors/parrots) or lightly under each wing (pigeon/passerine).

Reptiles: Spray on to cloth first then wipe over surface of reptile q7–14d until negative for ectoparasites. Beware of use in debilitated reptiles, those which have recently shed their skin and in small species where overdosage and toxicity may occur.

Amphibians, Fish: Not indicated.

NOTES

Firocoxib [25]
(Previcox) POM-V

Formulations: Oral: 57 mg, 227 mg tablets.

DOSES

Dogs: 5 mg/kg p.o. q24h, with or without food.

Dose rate	Patient bodyweight (kg)	mg/kg range	No. of tablets required	
			57 mg	*227 mg*
Dogs				
5 mg/ kg once daily	3–5.5	5.2–9.5	0.5	
	5.6–10	5.7–10.2	1	
	10.1–15	5.7–8.5	1.5	
	15.1–22	5.2–7.5		0.5
	22.1–45	5.0–10.3		1
	45.1–68	5.0–7.5		1.5
	68.1–90	5.0–6.7		2

Previcox (from datasheet)

Cats: Do not use.

NOTES

Fluids – composition of intravenous fluids [25, 26]

Fluid	Na+ (mmol/l)	K+ (mmol/l)	Ca2+ (mmol/l)	Cl− (mmol/l)	HCO3− (mmol/l)	Dext. (g/l)	Osmol. (mosml/l)
0.45% NaCl	77			77			155
0.9% NaCl	154			154			308
5% NaCl	856			856			1722
Ringer's	147	4	2	155			310
Lactated Ringer's (Hartmann's)	131	5	2	111	29 *		280
Darrow's	121	35		103	53 *		312
0.9% NaCl + 5.5% Dext.	154			154		50	560
0.18% NaCl + 4% Dext.	31			31		40	264
Duphalyte **		2.6	1	3.6		454	Unknown

Dext. = dextrose; Osmol. = osmolality. * Bicarbonate is present as lactate.
** Also contains a mixture of vitamins and small quantities of amino acids and 1.2 mmol/l of $MgSO_4$

NOTES

Fluids – estimating percentage of dehydration [7]

Clinical assessment findings	Estimated percentage dehydration
No clinical signs detectable	<5
Mild loss of skin elasticity, possible drying of oral mucous membranes	5–6
Definite reduction in skin elasticity, dry oral mucous membranes, eyes may start to look sunken, mild increase in capillary refill time	6–8
Skin tenting very obvious, dry oral mucous membranes, sunken eyes, signs of hypovolaemia (rapid heart rate, weak pulses, cool extremities)	8–10
Severe loss of skin elasticity, very dry mucous membranes, obvious signs of hypovolaemia, altered mentation with possible recumbency, anuria	10–12
Signs of shock, moribund, death imminent	12–15

Fluralaner [25]
(Bravecto) POM-V

Formulations: Chewable tablets 5 sizes delivering 25–56 mg fluralaner/kg.

DOSES

Dogs: 25–56 mg fluralaner/kg, every 3 months.

Cats: Do not use.

NOTES

Fly strike (myiasis) in the rabbit [23]

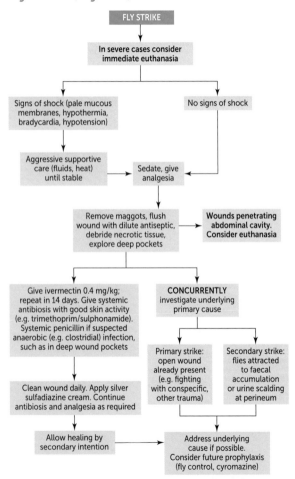

FLY STRIKE

In severe cases consider immediate euthanasia

Signs of shock (pale mucous membranes, hypothermia, bradycardia, hypotension)

No signs of shock

Aggressive supportive care (fluids, heat) until stable

Sedate, give analgesia

Remove maggots, flush wound with dilute antiseptic, debride necrotic tissue, explore deep pockets

Wounds penetrating abdominal cavity. Consider euthanasia

Give ivermectin 0.4 mg/kg; repeat in 14 days. Give systemic antibiosis with good skin activity (e.g. trimethoprim/sulphonamide). Systemic penicillin if suspected anaerobic (e.g. clostridial) infection, such as in deep wound pockets

CONCURRENTLY investigate underlying primary cause

Primary strike: open wound already present (e.g. fighting with conspecific, other trauma)

Secondary strike: flies attracted to faecal accumulation or urine scalding at perineum

Clean wound daily. Apply silver sulfadiazine cream. Continue antibiosis and analgesia as required

Allow healing by secondary intention

Address underlying cause if possible. Consider future prophylaxis (fly control, cyromazine)

Furosemide (Frusemide) [25, 26]

(Dimazon, Frusecare, Frusedale, Libeo, Frusol*) POM-V, POM

Formulations:

- Injectable: 50 mg/ml solution.
- Oral: 10 mg, 20 mg, 40 mg, 1gt tablets; 20 mg/5ml, 40 mg/5 ml, 50 mg/5ml sugar-free oral solution.

DOSES

Dogs, Cats:

- Acute, life-threatening congestive heart failure: 1–4 mg/kg i.v., i.m. q1–4h as required, based on improvement in respiratory rate and effort. Once clinical signs improve, increase dosing interval to q8–12h, monitor urea, creatinine and electrolytes, and start oral therapy once tolerated. Use lower end of dose range for cats and monitor response. Ensure no pleural effusion present.
- Chronic, congestive heart failure: 1–5 mg/kg p.o. q6–48h. Typical maintenance doses for mild to moderate CHF are 1–2 mg/kg p.o. q12–24h (dogs) and 1–2 mg/kg p.o. q12–48h (cats). The goal is to use the lowest dose of furosemide that effectively controls clinical signs. Doses in excess of 12 mg/kg/day are unlikely to be beneficial and warrant the addition of a different class of diuretic (e.g. thiazide) or transfer to alternative diuretic (e.g. torasemide) to control refractory failure. In patients with ascites, use of s.c. instead of p.o. furosemide can have a marked clinical benefit due to improved bioavailability.
- Hypercalciuric nephropathy: hydrate before therapy. Give 5 mg/kg bolus i.v., then begin 5 mg/kg/h infusion, or give 2–5 mg/kg i.v., s.c., p.o. q8–24h. Maintain hydration status and electrolyte balance with normal saline and added KCl. Furosemide generally reduces serum calcium levels by 0.5–1.5 mmol/l.
- Acute renal failure/uraemia: Replace fluid deficit and subsequently closely monitor fluid input and output. ⟫

Give furosemide at 2 mg/kg i.v. If no diuresis within 1 hour repeat dose at 2–4 mg/kg i.v. If no response within 1 hour give another dose at 2–4 mg/kg i.v. Alternatively, bolus dose with 1–2 mg/kg i.v. followed by constant rate infusion at 0.1–2mg/kg/h.

■ To promote diuresis in hyperkalaemic states: 2 mg/kg i.v. q6h.

Libeo (from datasheet)			
Dose rate	**Bodyweight (kg)**	**No. of tablets per dose, once or twice daily**	
		10 mg	*40 mg*
Dogs			
1–5 mg/kg	2–3.5	¼	Use Libeo 10 mg
	3.6–5	½	Use Libeo 10 mg
	5.1–7.5	¾	Use Libeo 10 mg
	7.6–10	1	¼
	10.1–12.5	1 ¼	Use Libeo 10 mg
	12.6–15	1 ½	Use Libeo 10 mg
	15.1–20	Use Libeo 40 mg	½
	20.1–30	Use Libeo 40 mg	¾
	30.1–40	Use Libeo 40 mg	1
	40.1–50	Use Libeo 40 mg	1¼

Mammals:

■ Primates, Sugar gliders: 1–4 mg/kg p.o., i.m., s.c. q8h
■ Hedgehogs: 2.5–5 mg/kg p.o., i.m., s.c. q8h
■ Ferrets: 1–4 mg/kg i.v., i.m., p.o. q8–12h
■ Rabbits: 1–4 mg/kg i.v., i.m. q4–6h initially; maintenance doses are often 1–2 mg/kg p.o. q8–24h

Rodents: 1–4 mg/kg s.c., i.m. q4–6h or 5–10 mg/kg s.c., i.m. q12h.

Birds: 0.1–6.0 mg/kg i.m., s.c., i.v. q6–24h.

Reptiles: 5 mg/kg i.m. q12–24h.

Amphibians: Not indicated.

Fish: No information available.

NOTES

Gabapentin (Gabapentinum) [25, 26]
(Neurontin*) POM

Formulations: Oral: 100 mg, 300 mg, 400 mg capsules; 600 mg, 800 mg film-coated tablets; 50 mg/ml solution.

DOSES

Dogs: 10–20 mg/kg p.o. q6-8h (starting dose; incremental dose increases are recommended).

Cats: 5–10 mg/kg p.o. q8–12h (starting dose; incremental dose increases are recommended).

Mammals:
- Ferrets: 3–5 mg/kg p.o. q8h
- Rabbits: 2–5 mg/kg p.o. q8h
- Hamsters: 50 mg/kg p.o. q24h
- Rats: 30 mg/kg p.o. q8h.

Birds: 10–11 mg/kg p.o. q12–24h.

Reptiles, Amphibians, Fish: No information available.

Gastric dilatation–volvulus (GDV) radiographic appearance [12]

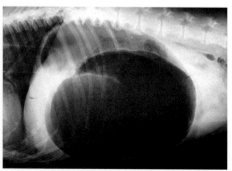

Right lateral radiograph of a dog with gastric dilatation–volvulus. Note the appearance of the pylorus in the craniodorsal abdomen as a gas-filled structure.

Gerbil biological data [21]

Lifespan (years)	2–3
Adult bodyweight (g)	Males: 46–131 Females: 50–55
Dentition	2 [I 1/1, C0/0, P0/0, M3/3] Only incisors open-rooted
Number of digits	Front: 5 Rear: 4
Rectal temperature (°C)	37.4–39
Heart rate (beats/min)	260–600
Respiratory rate (breaths/min)	85–160
Environmental temperature (°C)	18–22
Relative humidity (%)	45–50
Daily water intake	4–5 ml
Fluid therapy	40–60 ml/kg/24h
Diet	Largely granivorous
Food intake per day per animal (g)	5–7
Coprophagy/Caecotrophy?	Yes
Oestrous type	Continuous polyoestrous
Post-partum oestrus?	Yes (resulting in delayed implantation)
Age at puberty (months)	Males: 2–4.5 Females: 2–3
Gestation length (days)	23–46
Oestrous cycle (days)	4–6
Oestrus duration (hours)	12–18
Litter size	3–8
Birth weight (g)	2.5–3.5
Altricial/Precocial	Altricial
Eyes open (days)	16–21
Age at weaning (days)	21–28

Number of pairs of teats	4
Minimum breeding age (months)	2.5–3.5
Ratio for breeding (M:F)	1:1 Form monogamous lifelong pairs in captivity. Do not remove the male
Comments	Pseudopregnancy is common following infertile mating, lasting 14–16 days

Gestation periods in the bitch and queen [17]

- Bitch: 63 days from first mating (range 56–72 days).
- Queen: 65 days from first mating (range 52–74 days).

Glaucoma — common causes [12]

Primary

- Open angle/cleft
- Narrow/closed angle/cleft
- Pectinate ligament dysplasia/goniodysgenesis

Secondary

- Anterior uveitis[a]
- Lens luxation or subluxation
- Cataract
- Aphakic
- Hyphaema
- Intraocular neoplasia[a]
- Malignant/aqueous misdirection
- Melanocytic glaucoma
- Pigmentary and cystic glaucoma in Golden Retrievers
- Postoperative ocular hypertension
- Giant retinal tears

Congenital glaucoma

[a]Most common causes of glaucoma in cats.

Grape/raisin/sultana poisoning **(URGENT)**[1]

Also known as: *Vitis vinifera* fruits, grapevine fruits, currants

Description/exposure

Grapes and raisins are generally considered to be nephrotoxic to dogs. Ingestion of fruit, cooked products (e.g. baked goods, trail mix) or liquid sources (e.g. grape juice) is considered to result in toxicosis. There are no reports of toxicosis resulting from the ingestion of grapeseed extract.

Mechanism of action

Currently unknown.

Clinical presentation

Vomiting is often the first clinical sign. Lethargy, anorexia, abdominal pain, diarrhoea, dehydration, polyuria, polydipsia and uraemic breath may also be observed, typically >24 hours following exposure.

Diagnostics

Serum biochemistry (specifically a renal panel) and urinalysis (prior to fluid administration) should be performed on initial presentation. Repeat blood work to assess renal function should be performed every 24 hours whilst the patient is hospitalized.

Treatment

Although reports of toxic doses exist in the veterinary literature, more recently this type of toxicosis has been considered potentially idiosyncratic in some dogs. However, whilst not all dogs are clinically affected due to the idiosyncratic nature of the nephrotoxicant, aggressive gastrointestinal decontamination is still recommended in all patients. Induction of emesis can be attempted several hours after exposure as these products remain in the stomach for a prolonged period of time. Following the induction of emesis, one dose of an antiemetic and one dose of activated charcoal should be administered.

▣▶

Depending upon the success of emesis, intravenous fluids (4–10 ml/kg/h), antiemetic medication and gastroprotectants are recommended. Blood pressure monitoring, urine output and point-of-care blood work should be performed whilst the patient is hospitalized, as azotaemia with hypercalcaemia and hyperphosphataemia can be seen within 24 hours. Anecdotally, most dogs that are treated aggressively never develop acute kidney injury (AKI) and are successfully discharged from hospital several days after the initiation of treatment.

Prognosis

Dogs that develop AKI with oliguria or anuria have a poor to guarded prognosis.

NOTES

Guinea pig biological data [21]

Lifespan (years)	5–6
Adult bodyweight (g)	Males: 900–1200 Females: 700–900
Dentition	2 [I 1/1, C0/0, P1/1, M3/3]
Body temperature (°C)	37.2–39.5
Heart rate (beats/min)	230–380
Respiratory rate (breaths/min)	90–150
Tidal volume (ml/kg)	5–10
Food consumption	6 g per 100 g bodyweight/day
Water consumption	10 ml per 100 g bodyweight/day
Sexual maturity (months)	Males: 3–4 (600–700 g) Females: 2–3 (350–450 g)
Oestrous cycle	15–17 days; breeding duration of 18–48 months
Duration of oestrus (hours)	1–16
Gestation length (days)	59–72 (varies inversely with litter size, longer for small litters)
Parturition	Early morning. Farrowing: approximately 30 minutes; 5–10 minutes between pups
Post-partum oestrus	Yes
Litter size	1–6 (average 3–4)
Birth weight (g)	60–100; precocial; fully furred; ears open; teeth present
Eyes open (days)	Open at birth
Eat solid food (days)	May begin day after birth to nibble solid foods
Weaning (days)	14–21 (begin eating solid food and drinking water within 7 days)
Litters per year	Breeding colonies may have 3–4 litters per year
Commercial breeding life (years)	3–4
Chromosome number (diploid)	64

NOTES

Hamster biological data [21]

Lifespan (years)	1.5–2
Adult bodyweight (g)	Males: 87–130 Females: 95–130
Dentition	2 [I1/1 C0/0 P0/0 M3/3] Only incisors open-rooted
Number of digits	Front: 4 Rear: 5
Rectal temperature (°C)	36.2–37.5
Heart rate (beats/min)	300–470
Respiratory rate (breaths/min)	40–110
Environmental temperature (°C)	21–24
Relative humidity (%)	40–60
Daily water intake	10 ml/100g
Fluid therapy	102 ml/kg/24h
Diet	Omnivorous
Food intake per day per animal (g)	10–15
Coprophagy/Caecotrophy?	Yes
Oestrous type	Seasonal polyoestrous
Post-partum oestrus?	No
Age at puberty (months)	Males: 2 Females: 1.5
Gestation length (days)	Syrian: 16–18 Russian: 18–21 Chinese: 21–23 Roborovski: 23–30
Oestrous cycle (days)	4–5
Oestrus duration (hours)	8–26
Litter size	5–10
Birth weight (g)	1.5–3
Altricial/Precocial	Altricial

Eyes open (days)	12–14
Age at weaning (days)	19–21
Number of pairs of teats	6–7
Minimum breeding age (months)	2
Ratio for breeding (M:F)	1:1 Remove male after mating (except for Russian hamsters)
Comments	A vaginal discharge on day 2 of the oestrous cycle is normal and should not be confused with pyometra Cannibalism will occur if handled within 5 days of parturition Born with erupted incisors

NOTES

Head trauma – an approach to management [15]

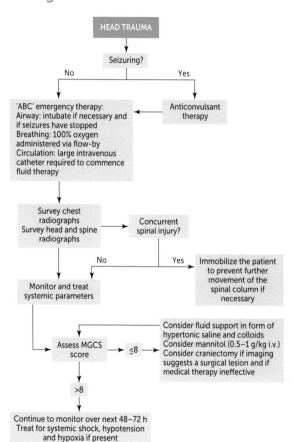

HEAD TRAUMA

Seizuring?

No → Yes

Yes → Anticonvulsant therapy

'ABC' emergency therapy:
Airway: intubate if necessary and if seizures have stopped
Breathing: 100% oxygen administered via flow-by
Circulation: large intravenous catheter required to commence fluid therapy

↓

Survey chest radiographs
Survey head and spine radiographs

→ Concurrent spinal injury?

No ↓

Yes → Immobilize the patient to prevent further movement of the spinal column if necessary

Monitor and treat systemic parameters

↓

Assess MGCS score

≤8 → Consider fluid support in form of hypertonic saline and colloids
Consider mannitol (0.5–1 g/kg i.v.)
Consider craniectomy if imaging suggests a surgical lesion and if medical therapy ineffective

>8 ↓

Continue to monitor over next 48–72 h
Treat for systemic shock, hypotension and hypoxia if present

MGCS = modified Glasgow coma scale.

See also Modified Glasgow coma scale

Heart murmur grading [20]

Grade	Characteristics on auscultation
1	Murmur barely audible
2	Murmur audible but less intense than normal cardiac sounds (S1/S2)
3	Murmur of equal intensity to S1/S2
4	Murmur of greater intensity than S1/S2
5	Loud murmur associated with precordial thrill
6	Murmur can be heard with stethoscope held away from chest wall

NOTES

Heart radiograph – 'clock face' analogy [8]

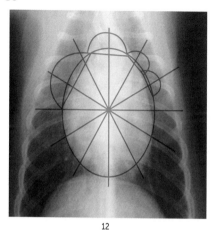

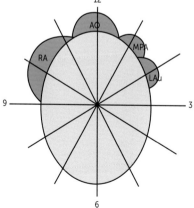

Clock face analogy of the cardiac silhouette on a DV or VD view. The location of dilatation of the left auricular appendage (LAu), main pulmonary artery (MPA), aorta (AO) and right atrium (RA) are shown.

Heart rate — reference values [8, 12, 21]

Species	Heart Rate (bpm)
Canine (adult)	70–160
Canine (puppy)	70–220
Feline (adult)	140–240[a]
Feline (kitten)	220–260
Chinchillas	200–350
Ferrets	200–250
Gerbils	260–600
Guinea Pigs	230–380
Hamsters	300–470
Mice	420–700
Rabbits	180–300
Rats	310–500

[a] In clinic; may be lower at home.

NOTES

Heart – vertebral heart score [19]

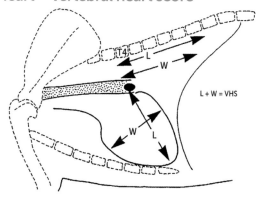

$$L + W = VHS$$

Technique to perform a VHS on a lateral radiograph. L = length of the cardiac silhouette; T4 = fourth thoracic vertebra; W = width of the cardiac silhouette. (Reproduced from Dennis *et al.* (2001) *Handbook of Small Animal Radiological Differential Diagnosis*, p.126. © Elsevier)

Dog mean value

9.7 ± 0.5 v
Have VHS values within the range of 8.5–10.5 v

Dog breed-specific values

Boxer: 11.6 ± 0.8 v
Cavalier King Charles Spaniel: 10.6 ± 0.5 v
Dobermann: 10.0 ± 0.6 v
German Shepherd Dog: 9.7 ± 0.7 v
Labrador Retriever: 10.8 ± 0.6 v
Whippet: 11.0 ± 0.5 v
Yorkshire Terrier: 9.7 ± 0.5 v

Puppies

Have VHS values within the same 8.5–10.5 v range

Cat mean value

7.5 ± 0.3 v on a lateral view
(The cardiac width on a DV/VD view is 3.4 ± 0.25 v if measured perpendicular to the long axis)

Normal vertebral heart score. v = vertebrae.

Hyperadrenocorticism [9]

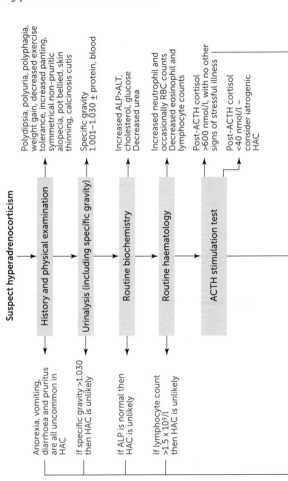

Suspect hyperadrenocorticism

History and physical examination → Polydipsia, polyuria, polyphagia, weight gain, decreased exercise tolerance, increased panting, symmetrical non-pruritic alopecia, pot bellied, skin thinning, calcinosis cutis

Anorexia, vomiting, diarrhoea and pruritus are all uncommon in HAC

Urinalysis (including specific gravity) → Specific gravity 1.001–1.030 ± protein, blood

If specific gravity >1.030 then HAC is unlikely

Routine biochemistry → Increased ALP>ALT, cholesterol, glucose. Decreased urea

If ALP is normal then HAC is unlikely

Routine haematology → Increased neutrophil and occasionally RBC counts. Decreased eosinophil and lymphocyte counts

If lymphocyte count >1.5 x 10⁹/l then HAC is unlikely

ACTH stimulation test → Post-ACTH cortisol >600 nmol/l, with no other signs of stressful illness

Post-ACTH cortisol <40 nmol/l – consider iatrogenic HAC

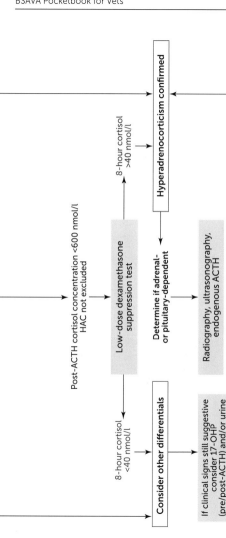

Post-ACTH cortisol concentration <600 nmol/l
HAC not excluded

Low-dose dexamethasone suppression test

8-hour cortisol >40 nmol/l → **Hyperadrenocorticism confirmed**

Determine if adrenal- or pituitary-dependent

Radiography, ultrasonography, endogenous ACTH

8-hour cortisol <40 nmol/l → **Consider other differentials**

If clinical signs still suggestive consider 17-OHP (pre/post-ACTH) and/or urine cortisol:creatinine ratio

A summary of the investigation of canine hyperadrenocorticism (HAC). It is not necessary to perform all these investigations in every case. Text in blue refers to typical features of HAC; text in red refers to uncommon findings.
ACTH = adrenocorticotropic hormone; ALP = alkaline phosphatase; ALT = alanine aminotransferase; 17-OHP = 17-hydroxyprogesterone; RBC = red blood cell.

Hypertension [2]

Risk category	Systolic blood pressure (mmHg)	Recommendation for starting treatment
Minimal	<150	■ Minimal to mild risk of developing target organ damage (TOD)
Mild	150–159	■ Limited evidence that anti-hypertensive medication required ■ May represent cases of 'white-coat' hypertension ■ Treatment should be considered if evidence of ocular or central nervous system TOD ■ Continued monitoring recommended ■ Target categories for patients treated with anti-hypertensive therapies
Moderate	160–179	■ Moderate risk for the development of TOD ■ Anti-hypertensive therapy recommended in patients with evidence of TOD or where concurrent clinical conditions associated with hypertension have been identified ■ Confirmation of hypertensive category status should be made on at least two occasions unless there is evidence of ocular or CNS TOD, when therapy will be required immediately ■ Patients in this category which have no evidence of TOD or clinical conditions associated with systemic hypertension should be monitored carefully to exclude white-coat hypertension before a diagnosis of idiopathic hypertension is made and long-term treatment started
Severe	180	■ The risk of development and progression of TOD is high ■ White coat hypertension is uncommon ■ Immediate anti-hypertensive therapy indicated if ocular or CNS TOD present otherwise confirmation of category status should be made on at least two occasions

ACVIM risk categories for systolic hypertension in dogs and cats.

NOTES

Hypoglycaemia [9]

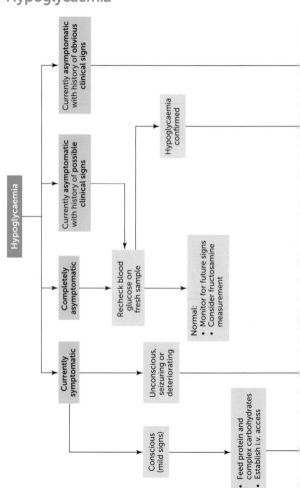

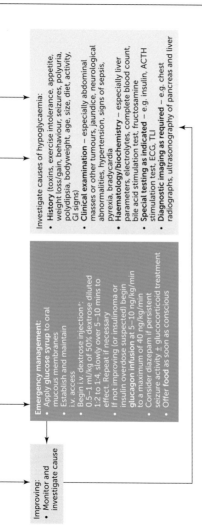

Investigate causes of hypoglycaemia:
- **History** (toxins, exercise intolerance, appetite, weight loss/gain, behaviour, seizures, polyuria, polydipsia, bodyweight, age, size, diet, activity, GI signs)
- **Clinical examination** – especially abdominal masses or other tumours, jaundice, neurological abnormalities, hypertension, signs of sepsis, pyrexia, bradycardia
- **Haematology/biochemistry** – especially liver parameters, electrolytes, complete blood count, bile acid stimulation test, fructosamine
- **Special testing as indicated** – e.g. insulin, ACTH stimulation test, ECG, TLI
- **Diagnostic imaging as required** – e.g. chest radiographs, ultrasonography of pancreas and liver

Emergency management:
- Apply **glucose syrup** to oral mucous membranes
- Establish and maintain i.v. access
- Begin i.v. dextrose injection[a]. 0.5–1 ml/kg of 50% dextrose diluted 1:2 to 1:4, slowly over 5–10 mins to effect. Repeat if necessary
- If not improving (or insulinoma or insulin overdose suspected) begin **glucagon infusion** at 5–10 ng/kg/min to a maximum of 40 ng/kg/min
- Consider diazepam if persistent seizure activity ± glucocorticoid treatment
- Offer **food** as soon as conscious

Improving:
- Monitor and investigate cause

A suggested diagnostic approach and emergency therapeutic approach to hypoglycaemia. [a] Avoid dextrose bolus in insulinoma cases if possible because this may lead to further insulin release. ACTH = adrenocorticotropic hormone; ECG = electrocardiography; GI = gastrointestinal; TLI = trypsin-like immunoreactivity.

NOTES

Imidacloprid [25, 26]

(Advantage, Advantix, Advocate, Bob Martin Double Action Dewormer, Clear Double Action Spot-on Solution, Clearspot, 4fleas and several combination products) POM-V, AVM-GSL

Formulations: Topical: 100 mg/ml imidacloprid either as sole agent or else in combination with moxidectin or permethrin (e.g. Advantix, Advocate, Prinovox and others) in spot-on pipettes of various sizes. Also used in collars impregnated with 1.25g/4.5g imidacloprid combined with flumethrin (Seresto). Numerous GSL and non-authorized formulations.

DOSES

Dogs: Fleas and ticks: 10 mg/kg topically every month. In dogs >40 kg the appropriate combination of pipettes should be applied. Collars should be replaced every 8 months.

Cats: Fleas: 10–20 mg/kg topically every month. Collars should be replaced every 8 months.

Mammals:
- Ferrets: 0.4 ml pipette q30d
- Rabbits: 0.4 ml, 0.8 ml pipettes (use the smaller size in rabbits <4 kg) or 0.125 ml/kg imidacloprid/permethrin formulation for fur mites (*Leporacus* spp.)
- Rabbits, Guinea pigs: 0.1 ml/kg imidacloprid/permethrin formulation
- Rodents: 20 mg/kg (equivalent to 0.2 ml/kg).

Birds: No information available.

Reptiles: Bearded dragons, Frillneck lizards: 0.2 ml/kg topically q14d for 3 treatments.

Amphibians, Fish: No information available.

NOTES

Insulin [25, 26]

(Caninsulin, Prozinc, Actrapid*, Humulin*, Hypurin*, Insulatard*, Lantus*) POM-V, POM

Formulations: Injectable: 40 IU/ml, 100 IU/ml suspensions (for s.c. injection) or 100 IU/ml solutions (for s.c., i.v. or i.m. injection). There are many preparations (including soluble) authorized for use in humans; however, veterinary authorized preparations (lente and PZI), when available, are preferential for both legal and clinical reasons.

Trade name	Species of insulin	Types available
Actrapid*	Human	Soluble (neutral)
Caninsulin	Porcine	Lente
Lantus*	Human	Glargine
Humulin*	Human	Soluble (neutral), Isophane
Hypurin*	Bovine	Soluble (neutral), Isophane, Lente, Protamine zinc insulin (PZI)
	Porcine	Soluble (neutral), Isophane
Insulatard*	Human or porcine	Isophane
Prozinc	Human	PZI

* = Not authorized for veterinary use.

DOSES

Dogs:

- Insulin-dependent diabetes mellitus (IDDM): Initially 0.25–0.5 IU/kg (dogs >25 kg) or 0.5–1 IU/kg (dogs <25 kg) of lente insulin s.c. q12h. Adjust dose and frequency of administration by monitoring clinical effect. Urine results, blood glucose and/or fructosamines may assist this process
- Diabetic ketoacidosis: 0.2 IU/kg soluble insulin i.m. initially followed by 0.1 IU/kg i.m. q1h. Alternatively i.v. infusions may be given at 0.025–0.06 IU/kg/h of soluble insulin. Run approximately 50 ml of i.v. solution

Type	Route	Onset	Peak effect in dog (hours)	Peak effect in cat (hours)	Duration of action in dog (hours)	Duration of action in cat (hours)
Soluble (neutral)	i.v.	Immediate	0.5–2	0.5–2	1–4	1–4
	i.m.	10–30 min	1–4	1–4	3–8	3–8
	s.c.	10–30 min	1–5	1–5	4–8	4–8
Semilente (amorphous IZS)	s.c.	30–60 min	1–5	1–5	4–10	4–10
Isophane (NPH)	s.c.	0.5–3 h	2–10	2–8	6–24	4–12
Lente (mixed IZS)	s.c.	30–60 min	2–10	2–8	8–24	6–14
Ultralente (crystalline IZS)	s.c.	2–8 h	4–16	4–16	8–28	8–24
PZI	s.c.	1–4 h	4–14	3–12	6–28	6–24
Glargine	s.c.	1–4 h	6–10	3–12	18–28	12–24

IZS = insulin zinc suspension; NPH = neutral protamine Hagedorn; PZI = protamine zinc insulin. Note that all times are approximate averages and insulin doses need to be adjusted for individual patients.

through tubing as insulin adheres to plastic; change insulin/saline solution q6h

■ Hyperkalaemic myocardial toxicity (not in hypoadrenocorticism): give a bolus of 0.5 IU/kg of soluble insulin i.v. followed by 2–3 g of dextrose/unit of insulin. Half the dextrose should be given as a bolus and the remainder administered i.v. over 4–6 hours.

Cats:

■ IDDM: Initially 0.25 IU/kg of lente insulin s.c. q12h or 0.2–0.4 IU/kg of PZI insulin s.c. q12h. Adjust dose and frequency of administration by monitoring clinical effect, urine results, blood glucose and/or fructosamine levels

■ Diabetic ketoacidosis: Doses as for dogs

■ Hyperkalaemic myocardial toxicity: Doses as for dogs.

Mammals:

■ Primates: Initially 0.25–0.5 IU/kg/day s.c. (NPH or lente insulin)

■ Ferrets: 0.5–1.0 IU/ferret s.c. q12h (lente) or 0.1 IU/ferret s.c. q24h (ultralente)

■ Chinchillas: 1 IU/kg s.c. q12h

■ Guinea pigs: 1–2 IU/kg s.c. q12h

■ Hamsters, Gerbils: 2 IU/animal s.c. q12h

■ Rats: 1–3 IU/rat s.c. q12h.

Birds: No information available.

Reptiles:

■ Chelonians, Snakes: 1–5 IU/kg i.m. q24–72h

■ Lizards: 5–10 IU/kg i.m. q24–72h; adjust doses according to serial glucose measurement.

Amphibians, Fish: No information available.

NOTES

Intraocular pressure (IOP) normal values[16, 28]

- **Dogs:** 10–25 mmHg.
- **Most other species:** 15–25 mmHg; the difference between fellow eyes should be less than 8 mmHg.

IRIS staging – acute kidney injury (AKI) [9]

Stage	Serum/plasma creatinine (µmol/l)	Clinical description
I	<140	Non-azotaemic or volume-responsive AKI Historical, clinical, laboratory or imaging evidence of renal injury Progressive non-azotaemic increase in creatinine ≥26 µmol/l (0.3 mg/dl) in 48 hours Measured oliguria (<1 ml/kg/h) or anuria over 6 hours
II	140–220	Mild AKI: historical, clinical, laboratory or imaging evidence of AKI and mild static or progressive azotaemia Progressive non-azotaemic increase in creatinine ≥26 µmol/l (0.3 mg/dl) in 48 hours Measured oliguria (<1 ml/kg/h) or anuria over 6 hours
III	221–439	Moderate to severe AKI: documented AKI and increasing severity of azotaemia and functional renal failure
IV	440–880	
V	>880	

Each stage is further sub-staged depending on whether the cat or dog is oligoanuric (O) or non-oliguric (NO) and on the requirement for renal replacement therapy (RRT).

NOTES

IRIS staging — chronic kidney disease (CKD) [9]

Stage	Plasma/serum creatinine (μmol/l)		Comments
	Dogs	*Cats*	
1	<125	<140	Non-azotaemic Some other renal abnormality present, such as persistent proteinuria or morphological abnormalities detected by imaging
2	125–180	140–250	Non-azotaemic to mildly azotaemic Clinical signs usually mild or absent
3	181–440	250–440	Mild to moderately azotaemic With or without clinical signs of uraemia
4	>440	>440	Severe azotaemia With or without clinical signs of uraemia
Sub-stage proteinuria	**UPCR**		
	Dogs	*Cats*	
Non-proteinuric (NP)	<0.2	<0.2	
Borderline proteinuric (BP)	0.2–0.5	0.2–0.4	
Proteinuric (P)	>0.5	>0.4	
Sub-stage blood pressure[a]			
Risk of end-organ damage	*Systolic (mmHg)*	*Diastolic (mmHg)*	
None (N)	<150	<95	
Low (L)	150–159	95–99	
Moderate (M)	160–179	100–119	
High (H)	>180	>120	

[a]Cut-offs are the same for dogs and cats. UPCR = urine protein:creatinine ratio.

Ivermectin [25, 26]

(Otimectin Vet, plus many others) POM-V, POM-VPS, ESPA

Formulations:

- Injectable: 1% w/v solution; Many different formulations authorized for use in farm animals and horses (e.g. Bimectin, Enovex, Ecomectin, Ivomec).
- Topical: 1 mg/g ear gel for cats; 100 µg/g, 800 µg/g spot-on tubes; 1 µg/ml, 10 µg/ml drops; 200 µg/ml spray (Xeno).

DOSES

Dogs:

- Generalized demodicosis: 300–600 µg (micrograms)/kg p.o. daily.
- Effective for sarcoptic mange (200–400 µg (micrograms)/kg p.o., s.c. q2w for 4–6 weeks) and cheyletiellosis (200–300 µg/kg p.o., s.c. q1–2w for 6–8 weeks) but other options (selamectin, moxidectin) are available.

Cats:

- Otoacariasis (*Otodectes cynotis* infestation): apply ear gel weekly for 3 weeks
- Generalized demodicosis: 300–600 µg (micrograms)/kg p.o. daily.

Mammals:

- Primates, Sugar gliders, Hedgehogs: 0.2–0.4 mg/kg s.c., p.o., repeat at 14 and 28 days (acariasis, nematodes)
- Small mammals: 0.2–0.5 mg/kg s.c., p.o. q7–14d
- Ferrets, Rabbits, Guinea pigs: apply 450 µg (micrograms)/kg (1 tube Xeno 450) topically
- Ferrets, small rodents <800 g: 50 µg (micrograms)/250 g (15 drops Xeno 50-mini) q7–14d.

Birds: 200 µg (micrograms)/kg i.m., s.c., p.o. q7–14d

- Raptors: capillariasis: 0.5–1 mg/kg i.m., p.o. q7–14d; *Serratospiculum*: 1 mg/kg p.o., i.m. q7–14d (moxidectin or doramectin may be given at same dose rates) ⟫⟫⟫

- Passerines and small psittacids: systemic dosing as above or 0.2 mg/kg applied topically to skin using 0.02% solution (in propylene glycol) q7–14d
- Pigeons: 0.5 ml applied topically to bare skin using 0.02% solution q7–14d
- Ornamental birds: mites and lice: 1 drop/50 g bodyweight weekly for 3 weeks.

Reptiles: 0.2 mg/kg s.c., p.o. once, repeat in 10–14 days until negative for parasites; may use as environmental control for snake mites (*Ophionyssus natricis*) at dilution of 5 mg/l water sprayed in tank q7–10d (if pre-mix ivermectin with propylene glycol this facilitates mixing with water)

- Chelonians: *do not use*.

Amphibians: 0.2–0.4 mg/kg p.o. q14d or 2 mg/kg topically, repeat in 14–21 days or 10 mg/l for 60 minute bath, repeat in 14 days.

Fish: No information available.

NOTES

NOTES

Ketamine [25, 26]

(Anesketin, Ketaset injection, Ketavet, Narketan-10, Vetalar-V) POM-V CD SCHEDULE 2

Formulations: Injectable: 100 mg/ml solution.

DOSES

Dogs:

- Perioperative analgesia: Intraoperatively: 10 µg (micrograms)/kg/min, postoperatively: 2–5 µg/kg/min, both preceded by a 250–500 µg/kg loading dose. There is some evidence to suggest that a 10 µg/kg/min dose may be too low to provide adequate analgesia continuously, although other evidence-based dose recommendations are lacking.
- Induction of anaesthesia (combined with diazepam or midazolam) as part of a volatile anaesthetic technique: 2 mg/kg i.v.
- Induction of general anaesthesia combined with medetomidine or dexmedetomidine to provide a total injectable combination: ketamine (5–7 mg/kg i.m.) combined with medetomidine (40 µg (micrograms)/kg i.m.) or dexmedetomidine (20 µg/kg i.m.).

Cats:

- General anaesthesia: combinations of ketamine (5–7.5 mg/kg i.m.) combined with medetomidine (80 µg (micrograms)/kg i.m.) or dexmedetomidine (40 µg/kg i.m.) will provide 20–30 min general anaesthesia. Reduce the doses of both drugs when given i.v.
- Perioperative analgesia: Doses are the same as those for dogs.

Mammals:

- Ferrets: 10–30 mg/kg i.m., s.c. alone gives immobilization and some analgesia but there is poor muscle relaxation and prolonged recovery. For general anaesthesia, sedate first and then induce with isoflurane or sevoflurane. Alternatively, combinations of ketamine (10–15 mg/kg) with medetomidine

(0.08–0.1 mg/kg i.m., s.c.) or dexmedetomidine (0.04–0.05 mg/kg i.m., s.c.) will provide a short period of heavy sedation or general anaesthesia in most ferrets. The duration and depth of anaesthesia is increased by the addition of butorphanol at 0.2–0.4 mg/kg i.m., s.c. or buprenorphine at 0.02 mg/kg i.m., s.c. which also provides analgesia. For perioperative/postoperative analgesia: 0.3–1.2 mg/kg/h CRI following 2–5 mg/kg i.v. loading dose. For postoperative analgesia: 0.1–0.4 mg/kg/h CRI.

- Rabbits: 15–30 mg/kg i.m., s.c. alone gives moderate to heavy sedation with some analgesia but there is poor muscle relaxation and prolonged recovery. Alternatively, 5 mg/kg i.v. or 10–15 mg/kg i.m., s.c. in combination with medetomidine (0.05–0.1 mg/kg i.v., 0.1–0.3 mg/kg s.c., i.m.) or dexmedetomidine (0.025–0.05 mg/kg i.v. or 0.05–0.15 mg/kg s.c., i.m.) and butorphanol (0.1–0.5 mg/kg i.v., s.c., i.m.) or buprenorphine (0.02–0.05 mg/kg i.m., i.v., s.c.) will give a short duration of heavy sedation or anaesthesia in most rabbits. Intravenous combinations are ideally given incrementally to effect.

- Guinea pigs: 10–50 mg/kg i.m., s.c. will provide immobilization, with little muscle relaxation and some analgesia, however it is suggested to use the lower end of the dose range to sedate first and then induce with isoflurane or sevoflurane; alternatively, a combination of ketamine (3–5 mg/kg i.m., s.c.) with medetomidine (0.10 mg/kg i.m., s.c.) or dexmedetomidine (0.05 mg/kg i.m., s.c.) will provide a short period of anaesthesia.

- Other rodents and small mammals: 10–50 mg/kg i.m., s.c. will provide immobilization, however it is suggested to use the lower end of the dose range and to induce anaesthesia with isoflurane or sevoflurane or use in combination with other agents (e.g. 5 mg/kg i.m., i.v., s.c. ketamine with 0.05–0.1 mg/kg i.m., i.v. medetomidine).

Birds: Largely superseded by gaseous anaesthesia.

Reptiles: Variable sedation and poor muscle relaxation if used alone. Prolonged recovery at higher dose rates. Usually combined with alpha-2 agonists and/or opioids/midazolam to provide deep sedation/light anaesthesia.

- Chelonians: 20–60 mg/kg i.m., i.v.
- Lizards: 25–60 mg/kg i.m., i.v.
- Snakes: 20–80 mg/kg i.m., i.v.

All doses given alone.

Amphibians: 50–150 mg/kg s.c., i.m. alone has long induction and recovery times. It is suggested to use 20–40 mg/kg i.m. in combination with diazepam at 0.2–0.4 mg/kg i.m.

Fish: 66–88 mg/kg i.m. alone or 1–2 mg/kg i.m. ketamine in combination with 0.05–0.1 mg/kg i.m. medetomidine, reversed with 0.2 mg/kg i.m. atipamezole.

See also Sedation combinations

Ketamine CRI for a 2 kg rabbit undergoing surgery [23]

- Fluid requirement is 10 ml/kg/h; 2 × 10 ml = 20 ml is required per hour.
- Ketamine requirement is 0.2 mg/kg/h. Concentration is 100 mg/ml.
- 0.2 × 2/100 = 0.004 ml is required per hour. This is added to 20 ml of fluid therapy and the syringe driver set to deliver 20 ml/h.

Kidney ***see*** IRIS staging

NOTES

Lactulose [25, 26]

(Duphalac*, Lactugal*, Lactulose*, Laevolac*) P

Formulations: Oral: 3.3 g/5 ml lactulose in a syrup base. Lactugal is equivalent to 62.0–74.0% w/v of lactulose.

DOSES

Dogs:
- Constipation: 0.5–1.0 ml/kg p.o. q8–12h. Monitor and adjust therapy to produce 2 or 3 soft stools per day.
- Acute hepatic encephalopathy: 18–20 ml/kg of a solution comprising 3 parts lactulose to 7 parts water per rectum as a retention enema for 4–8 h.
- Chronic hepatic encephalopathy: 0.5–1.0 ml/kg p.o. q8–12h. Monitor and adjust therapy to produce 2 or 3 soft stools per day.

Cats: Constipation and chronic hepatic encephalopathy: 0.5–5 ml p.o. q8–12h. Monitor and adjust therapy to produce 2 or 3 soft stools per day.

Mammals:
- Ferrets: 0.15–0.75 ml/kg p.o. q12h
- Rodents: 0.5 ml/kg p.o. q12h.

Birds: Appetite stimulant, hepatic encephalopathy: 0.2–1 ml/kg p.o. q8–12h.

Reptiles: 0.5 ml/kg p.o. q24h.

Amphibians, Fish: No information available.

Levothyroxine (T4, L-Thyroxine) [25, 26]

(Leventa, Soloxine, Thyforon) POM-V

Formulations: Oral: 0.1 mg, 0.2 mg, 0.3 mg, 0.5 mg, 0.8 mg tablets; 1 mg/ml solution.

DOSES

Dogs, Cats: Hypothyroidism 0.02–0.04 mg/kg/day. Alternatively, dose at 0.5 mg/m^2 body surface area daily. Dose given with food once or divided twice a day. Monitor serum T4 levels pre-dosing and 4–8 hours after dosing.

Dose rate	Patient bodyweight (kg)	Volume required (ml)			
		Dosage 10 µg/kg	Dosage 20 µg/kg	Dosage 30 µg/kg	Dosage 40 µg/kg
Dogs					
Recommended starting dose of 20 µg/kg once daily	5	0.05	0.10	0.15	0.20
	10	0.10	0.20	0.30	0.40
	15	0.15	0.30	0.45	0.60
	20	0.20	0.40	0.60	0.80
	25	0.25	0.50	0.75	1.00
	30	0.30	0.60	0.90	1.20
	35	0.35	0.70	1.05	1.40
	40	0.40	0.80	1.20	1.60
	45	0.45	0.90	1.35	1.80
	50	0.50	1.00	1.50	2.00

Leventa (from datasheet)

Mammals: Rodents: 5 µg (micrograms)/kg p.o. q12h.

Birds: 0.02 mg/kg p.o. q12–24h. Dissolve 1 mg in 28.4 ml water and give 0.4–0.5 ml/kg q12–24h.

Reptiles: Tortoises: 0.02 mg/kg p.o. q24–48h has been reported for the management of hypothyroidism in a Galapagos tortoise and an African spurred tortoise.

Amphibians, Fish: No information available.

NOTES

Lidocaine (Lignocaine) [25, 26]
(EMLA, Intubeaze, Lignadrin, Lignol, Locaine, Locovetic, Lidoderm*) POM-V

Formulations:
- Injectable: 1%, 2% solutions (some contain adrenaline).
- Topical: 2% solution (Intubeaze), 4% solution (Xylocaine); 2.5% cream with prilocaine (EMLA); 5% transdermal patches (Lidoderm).

DOSES

Note: 1 mg/kg is 0.05 ml/kg of a 2% solution.

Dogs:
- Local anaesthesia: Apply to the affected area with a small gauge needle to an appropriate volume. Total dose that should be injected is 4 mg/kg.
- Oesophagitis: 2 mg/kg p.o. q4–6h.
- Topical: Apply thick layer of cream to the skin and cover with a bandage for 45–60 min prior to venepuncture.
- Intraoperative analgesia given by constant rate infusion: 1 mg/kg loading dose (given slowly over 10–15 min) followed by 20–50 µg (micrograms)/kg/min. Postoperatively, similar dose rates can be used but should be adjusted according to pain assessment and be aware of the likelihood of accumulation allowing an empirical reduction in dose rate over time.
- Ventricular arrhythmias: 2–8 mg/kg i.v. in 2 mg/kg boluses followed by a constant rate i.v. infusion of 0.025–0.1 mg/kg/min.

Cats:
- Local anaesthesia, topical, oesophagitis: Doses as for dogs. Avoid systemic lidocaine for analgesia in cats due to the risk of drug accumulation, toxicity and negative haemodynamic effects.
- Ventricular arrhythmias: 0.25–2.0 mg/kg i.v. slowly in 0.25–0.5 mg/kg boluses followed by a constant rate i.v. infusion of 0.01–0.04 mg/kg/min.

Mammals: Local anaesthesia: apply to the affected area with a small gauge needle to an appropriate volume. Total dose that should be injected should not exceed 4 mg/kg (ideally 1–3 mg/kg).

- Rabbits: 0.3 ml/kg for epidural anaesthesia or 1–2 mg/ml i.v. bolus for cardiac arrhythmias or 2–4 mg/ml intratracheal for cardiac arrhythmias.
- Topical: apply thick layer of cream to the skin and cover with a bandage for 45–60 min prior to venepuncture.

Birds: <4 mg/kg as local infusion/nerve block. Do not use preparations with adrenaline.

Reptiles, Amphibians: 1–2 mg/kg as local infusion/nerve block. Do not exceed 5 mg/kg total dose per animal due to cardiotoxic side effects.

Fish: No information available.

Lipid infusions [25]

(ClinOleic*, Intralipid*, Ivelip*, Lipidem*, Lipofundin*, Omegaven*) POM

Formulations: Injectable: 10% solution contains soya oil emulsion, glycerol, purified egg phospholipids and phosphate (15 mmol/l) for i.v. use only. Contains 2 kcal/ml (8.4 kJ/ml), 268 mOsm/l. Other human products available and vary in composition.

DOSES

Dogs: The amount required will be governed by the patient's physiological status and whether partial or total parenteral nutrition is provided. Generally lipid infusions are used to supply 30% (partial peripheral) to 40–60% of energy requirements.

Cats: The amount required will be governed by the patient's physiological status and its tolerance of lipids. Generally, peripheral parenteral nutrition is provided by amino acids in cats and lipids are used as an energy source in a nutrient admixture for infusion through central venous access (total parenteral nutrition) to supply 40–60% of energy requirements.

⟼

Dogs, Cats: For treatment of lipid-soluble toxicosis such as ivermectin or moxidectin toxicosis, administer 1.5–5 ml/kg i.v. of 20% lipid solution as bolus, followed by 0.25–0.50 ml/kg/min i.v. infusion for 30–60 min. Boluses of 1.5 ml/kg can be repeated. Infusions of 0.5 ml/kg/min can be administered for a maximum of 24 hours.

Lufenuron [25, 26]

(Program, Program plus) POM-V

Formulations:

- Oral: 67.8 mg, 204.9 mg, 409.8 mg tablets (Program); 133 mg, 266 mg suspension (Program for cats). Also combined with 46 mg, 115 mg, 230 mg, 460 mg lufenuron with milbemycin (ratio of 20 mg lufenuron: 1 mg milbemycin) tablets (Program plus, Protect)
- Injectable: 40 mg, 80 mg prefilled syringes containing 100 mg/ml suspension (Program).

DOSES

Dogs: Fleas: 10 mg/kg p.o., s.c. q1month (equivalent to a dose of 0.5 mg/kg milbemycin in combined preparations).

Cats: Fleas: 10 mg/kg s.c. q6months or 30 mg/kg p.o. q1month.

Mammals:
- Ferrets: 30–45 mg/kg p.o. q1month
- Rabbits: 30 mg/kg p.o. q30d.

Birds, Reptiles, Amphibians: No information available.

Fish: 0.1 mg/l by immersion as required.

NOTES

NOTES

Maropitant [25]
(Cerenia) POM-V

Formulations:
- Injectable: 10 mg/ml solution.
- Oral: 16 mg, 24 mg, 60 mg, 160 mg tablets.

DOSES

Dogs:
- Vomiting: 1 mg/kg s.c. q24h or 2 mg/kg p.o. q24h.
- Motion sickness: tablets at a dose rate of 8 mg/kg q24h for a maximum of 2 days.
- Prevention of chemotherapy-induced emesis and motion sickness. 1 mg/kg s.c. q24h or 2 mg/kg p.o. q24h, given at least 1 hour in advance.

Cerenia (from datasheet)					
Dose rate	**Patient bodyweight (kg)**	**No. of tablets required**			
		16 mg	*24 mg*	*60 mg*	*160 mg*
Dogs					
Treatment and prevention of vomiting (except motion sickness): 2 mg/kg once daily (Not to be used in dogs <8 weeks old)	3.0–4.0*	½			
	4.1–8.0	1			
	8.1–12.0		1		
	12.1–24.0		2		
	24.1–30.0			1	
	30.1–60.0			2	
Prevention of motion sickness only: 8 mg/kg once daily (Not to be used in dogs <16 weeks old)	1.0–1.5		½		
	1.6–2.0	1			
	2.1–3.0		1		
	3.1–4.0	2			
	4.1–6.0		2		
	6.1–7.5			1	
	7.6–10.0				½
	10.1–15.0			2	
	15.1–20.0				1
	20.1–30.0				1½
	30.1–40.0				2
	40.1–60.0				3

* Correct dose for dogs <3 kg cannot be accurately achieved

Cats: Vomiting: 1 mg/kg s.c. or p.o q24h.

Medetomidine [25, 26]

(Domitor, Dorbene, Dormilan, Medetor, Sedastart, Sedator, Sededorm) POM-V

Formulations: Injectable: 1 mg/ml solution.

DOSES

Dogs, Cats: Premedication: 5–20 μg (micrograms)/kg i.v., i.m, s.c. in combination with an opioid. Use lower end of dose range i.v. Doses of 1–2 μg/kg i.v. can be used to manage excitation in the recovery period, although following administration animals must be monitored carefully. A continuous rate infusion of 2–4 μg/kg/h can be used to provide perioperative analgesia and rousable sedation, particularly when administered as an adjunct to opioid-mediated analgesia.

Mammals:
- Ferrets: 80–100 μg (micrograms)/kg i.m., s.c. in combination with an opioid and ketamine
- Rabbits: 100–300 μg (micrograms)/kg i.v., i.m., s.c. (use the lower end of the dose range when giving i.v.) in combination with an opioid and ketamine
- Rodents and other small mammals: Doses from 100–200 μg (micrograms)/kg i.p., i.m., s.c. in combination with ketamine and/or opioids or as premedication prior to induction with a volatile anaesthetic.

Birds: See the BSAVA Small Animal Formulary – Part B: Exotic Pets.

Reptiles: 100–200 μg (micrograms)/kg i.m; may be combined with ketamine and/or opioids or midazolam to provide deep sedation/light anaesthesia
- Desert tortoises: 150 μg (micrograms)/kg i.m.

Amphibians: No information available.

Fish: 0.01–0.05 mg/kg combined with 1–2 mg/kg ketamine i.m.

See also Sedation combinations

Meloxicam [25, 26]

(Inflacam, Loxicom, Meloxidyl, Meloxivet, Metacam, Revitacam, Rheumocam) POM-V

Formulations:

- Oral: 0.5 mg/ml suspension for cats, 1.5 mg/ml oral suspension for dogs; 1.0 mg, 2.5 mg tablets for dogs.
- Injectable: 2 mg/ml solution for cats, 5 mg/ml solution.

DOSES

Dogs: Initial dose is 0.2 mg/kg s.c., p.o.; if given as a single preoperative injection effects last for 24 hours. Can be followed by a maintenance dose of 0.1 mg/kg p.o q24h.

Metacam Chewable Tablets for Dogs (from datasheet)				
Dose rate	Patient bodyweight (kg)	No. of tablets per dose, once daily		mg/kg
		1 mg	2.5 mg	
Dogs				
0.1 mg/kg (maintenance dose)	4.0–7.0	½		0.13–0.1
	7.1–10.0	1		0.14–0.1
	10.1–15.0	1½		0.15–0.1
	15.1–20.0	2		0.13–0.1
	20.1–25.0		1	0.12–0.1
	25.1–35.0		1½	0.15–0.1
	35.1–50.0		2	0.14–0.1

Cats:

- Initial injectable dose is 0.2 mg/kg s.c.; if given as a single preoperative injection effects last for 24 hours. To continue treatment for up to 5 days, may be followed 24 hours later by the oral suspension for cats at a dosage of 0.05 mg/kg p.o.
- Postoperative pain/inflammation: single injection of 0.3 mg/kg s.c. has been shown to be safe and efficacious. It is not recommended to follow this with oral meloxicam 24 hours later.

■ Chronic pain: initial oral dose is 0.1 mg/kg p.o. q24h, which can be followed by a maintenance dose of 0.05 mg/kg p.o q24h. Treatment should be discontinued after 14 days if no clinical improvement is apparent.

Mammals:
■ Ferrets: 0.2 mg/kg p.o., s.c., i.m. q24h
■ Rabbits: 0.3–0.6 mg/kg s.c., p.o. q24h; studies have shown that rabbits may require a dose exceeding 0.3 mg/kg q24h to achieve optimal plasma levels of meloxicam over a 24-hour interval and doses of 1.5 mg/kg s.c., p.o. are well tolerated for 5 days
■ Rats: 1–2 mg/kg s.c., p.o. q24h
■ Mice: 2 mg/kg s.c. p.o. q24h
■ Other mammals: 0.2 mg/kg p.o., s.c. q24h has been suggested.

Birds: 0.5–1.0 mg/kg i.m., p.o. q12–24h.

Reptiles: 0.1–0.5 mg/kg p.o., s.c., i.m. has been suggested
■ Bearded dragons: 0.4 mg/kg i.m. q24h
■ Green iguanas: 0.2 mg/kg i.v., p.o. q24h.

Amphibians: 0.4 mg/kg p.o., s.c., intracoelomic q24h.

Fish: No information available.

NOTES

Metaflumizone [25]

(Promeris, Promeris Duo) POM-V

Formulations: Topical: 200 mg/ml spot-on pipettes of various sizes (Promeris); 150 mg/ml metaflumizone + 150 mg/ml amitraz in various sizes (Promeris Duo).

DOSES

Dogs: 40 mg/kg applied topically once for lice (amitraz-containing product) or every 4 weeks for fleas (both products) and ticks (amitraz-containing product).

Cats: 40 mg/kg applied topically every 4 weeks for fleas. Do not use Promeris Duo in cats.

Methadone [25]

(Comfortan) POM-V CD SCHEDULE 2

Formulations:
- Injectable: 10 mg/ml solution (generic preservative-free preparations are also available).
- Oral: 10 mg tablets.

DOSES

Dogs: Analgesia: 0.1–0.5 mg/kg i.m. or 0.1–0.3 mg/kg i.v. prn.

Cats:
- Analgesia: 0.1–0.5 mg/kg i.m. or 0.1–0.3 mg/kg i.v. prn.
- Doses in the range of 0.6 mg/kg are appropriate for oral transmucosal administration in cats.

Mammals: Analgesia: Rabbits: 0.3–0.7 mg/kg slow i.v., i.m.

Birds, Reptiles, Amphibians, Fish: No information available.

See also Sedation combinations

NOTES

Methimazole (Thiamazole) [25, 26]
(Felimazole, Thyronorm) POM-V

Formulations: Oral: 1.25 mg, 2.5 mg, 5 mg tablets; 5 mg/ml solution. Also available as a transdermal formulation on a named patient basis.

DOSES

Dogs: Hyperthyroidism: 2.5–5 mg/dog p.o. q12h depending on size.

Cats: Hyperthyroidism: 2.5 mg/cat p.o. q12h. Apply transdermal gel to pinna.

Mammals: Guinea pigs: 0.5–2.0 mg/kg p.o. q24h.

Reptiles: Snakes: 2 mg/kg p.o. q24h for 30 days.

Birds, Amphibians, Fish: No information available.

Methoprene (*S*-Methoprene) [25]
(Acclaim spray, Broadline, Certifect, Frontline Combo/Plus, R.I.P. fleas, Staykill) POM-V, NFA-VPS, GSL

Formulations:
- Topical: 9% *S*-methoprene with fipronil in spot-on pipettes of various sizes (e.g. Frontline Combo/Plus) also combination with additonal amitraz (Certifect), and a combination with eprinomectin, fipronil, praziquantel (Broadline).
- Environmental: *S*-methoprene with permethrin (Acclaim) or tetramethrine + permethrin (R.I.P. Fleas) household sprays.

DOSES

Dogs, Cats: Fleas: 1 pipette per animal monthly according to bodyweight.

NOTES

Metoclopramide [25, 26]
(Emeprid, Vomend, Metomotyl, Maxolon*,
Metoclopramide*) POM-V, POM

Formulations:
- Injectable: 5 mg/ml solution in 10 ml multi-dose vial or clear glass ampoules, 2.5 mg/ml solution.
- Oral: 10 mg tablet; 15 mg capsule; 1 mg/ml solution.

DOSES

Dogs, Cats: 0.25–0.5 mg/kg i.v., i.m., s.c., p.o. q12h or 0.17–0.33 mg/kg i.v., i.m., s.c., p.o. q8h or 1–2 mg/kg i.v. over 24 hours as a constant rate infusion.

Mammals:
- Primates, Hedgehogs: 0.2–0.5 mg/kg i.m., p.o. q8h
- Sugar gliders: 0.05–0.1 mg/kg i.v., i.m., s.c., p.o. q6–12h
- Ferrets, Rabbits, Guinea pigs: 0.5–1 mg/kg s.c., p.o. q6–12h.

Birds: 0.3–2.0 mg/kg p.o., i.m. q8–24h.

Reptiles: 0.05–1 mg/kg p.o., i.m. q24h. Higher doses may be needed in Desert tortoises.

Amphibians, Fish: No information available.

NOTES

Metronidazole [25, 26]
(Metrobactin, Stomorgyl, Flagyl*, Metrolyl*, Metronidazole*)
POM-V, POM

Formulations:

- Injectable: 5 mg/ml i.v. infusion.
- Oral: 200 mg, 250 mg, 400 mg, 500 mg tablets; 25 mg metronidazole + 46.9 mg spiramycin tablets, 125 mg metronidazole + 234.4 mg spiramycin tablets, 250 mg metronidazole + 469 mg spiramycin tablets (Stomorgyl 2, 10 and 20, respectively); 40 mg/ml oral solution.

DOSES

Dogs and Cats:

- Metronidazole: 25 mg/kg p.o. q12h or 50 mg/kg p.o. q24h. 10–15 mg/kg s.c., slow i.v. infusion q12h. Injectable solution may be given intrapleurally to treat empyema.
- Stomorgyl: 12.5 mg metronidazole + 23.4 mg spiramycin/kg p.o. (equivalent to 1 tablet/2 kg of Stomorgyl 2, 1 tablet/10 kg of Stomorgyl 10 and 1 tablet/20 kg of Stomorgyl 20) q24h for 5–10 days.

Metrobactin (from datasheet)			
Dose rate	Bodyweight (kg)	No. of tablets daily	
		250 mg	500 mg
Dogs and cats			
50 mg/kg q24h	1–1.25	¼	
	>1.25–2.5	½	
	>2.5–3.75	¾	
	>3.75–5	1	½
	>5–7.5	1½	¾
	>7.5–10	2	1
	>10–15	3	1½
	>15–20	4	2
	>20–25		2½
	>25–30		3
	>30–35		3½
	>35–40		4

Mammals:
- Primates: 25 mg/kg p.o. q12h
- Sugar gliders: 80 mg/kg p.o. q24h
- Hedgehogs: 20 mg/kg p.o. q12h
- Ferrets: 15–20 mg/kg p.o q12h or 50–75 mg/kg p.o. q24h for 14 days with clarithromycin and omeprazole for *Helicobacter*
- Rabbits, Chinchillas, Guinea pigs: 10–20 mg/kg p.o. q12h or 40 mg/kg p.o. q24h; 50 mg/kg p.o. q12h for 5 days may be required for giardiasis in chinchillas but use with caution
- Rats, Mice: 20 mg/kg s.c. q24h
- Other rodents: 20–40 mg/kg p.o. q24h.

Birds:
- Raptors: 50 mg/kg p.o. q24h for 5 days
- Pigeons: 40–50 mg/kg p.o. q24h for 5–7 days or 100 mg/kg p.o. q48h for 3 doses or 200 mg/kg p.o. once
- Parrots: 30 mg/kg p.o. q12h
- Passerines: 50 mg/kg p.o. q12h or 200 mg/l water daily for 7 days.

Reptiles:
- Anaerobic bacterial infections: Green iguanas, Snakes (Elaphe species): 20 mg/kg p.o. q24–48h.
- Protozoal infections: Chelonians: 100–125 mg/kg p.o., repeat after 14 days (use lower doses of 50 mg/kg p.o. q24h for 3–5 days for severe infections); Chameleons: 40–60 mg/kg p.o., repeat after 14 days; Milksnakes: 40 mg/kg p.o., repeat after 14 days; Other snakes: 100 mg/kg p.o., repeat after 14 days.

Amphibians: 50 mg/kg p.o. q24h for 3–5 days or 50 mg/l as a bath for up to 24 hours.

Fish: 25 mg/l by immersion q48h for 3 doses or 100 mg/kg p.o. q24h for 3 days.

Milbemycin [25, 26]

(Milbemax, Nexguard Spectra, Program plus, Trifexis) POM-V

Formulations: Oral: 2.5 mg and 12.5 mg milbemycin with praziquantel tablets (Milbemax for dogs and several others); 4 mg and 16 mg with praziquantel tablets (Milbemax for cats); 2.3 mg, 5.75 mg, 11.5 mg, 23 mg milbemycin with lufenuron (ratio 20 mg lufeneron: 1 mg milbemycin) tablets (Program plus); 1.875 mg, 3.75 mg, 7.5 mg, 15 mg, 30 mg milbemycin with afoxolaner (Nexguard Spectra); 4.5 mg, 7.1 mg, 11.1 mg, 17.4 mg, 27 mg milbemycin with spinosad (Trifexis).

DOSES

Dogs: Nematodes: 0.5 mg milbemycin/kg p.o. q30d. For *Angiostrongylus vasorum*: administer same dose 4 times at weekly intervals.

Cats: Nematodes: 2 mg milbemycin/kg p.o. q30d.

Milbemax (from datasheet)			
Dose rate	Patient bodyweight (kg)	No. of tablets required	
		MILBEMAX tablets for small dogs and puppies/small cats and kittens, respectively	MILBEMAX tablets for dogs/cats, respectively
Dogs			
0.5 mg milbemycin oxime and 5 mg praziquantel per kg	1–5	1	
	5–25		1
	>25–50		2
	>50–75		3
Cats			
2 mg milbemycin oxime and 5 mg praziquantel per kg	0.5–1	½	
	>1–2	1	
	2–4		½
	>4–8		1
	>8–12		1½

Mammals: Ferrets: 1.15–2.33 mg/kg p.o. q30d.

Birds, Reptiles, Amphibians, Fish: No information available.

Modified Glasgow coma scale (MGCS) [15]

Motor activity	Score
Normal gait, normal spinal reflexes	6
Hemiparesis, tetraparesis or decerebrate rigidity	5
Recumbent, intermittent extensor rigidity	4
Recumbent, constant extensor rigidity	3
Recumbent, constant extensor rigidity with opisthotonus	2
Recumbent, hypotonia of muscles, depressed or absent spinal reflexes	1
Brainstem reflexes	
Normal pupillary light reflexes and oculocephalic reflexes	6
Slow pupillary light reflexes and normal to reduced oculocephalic reflexes	5
Bilateral unresponsive miosis with normal to reduced oculocephalic reflexes	4
Pinpoint pupils with reduced to absent oculocephalic reflexes	3
Unilateral, unresponsive mydriasis with reduced to absent oculocephalic reflexes	2
Bilateral, unresponsive mydriasis with reduced to absent oculocephalic reflexes	1
Level of consciousness	
Occasional periods of alertness and responsive to environment	6
Depression or delirium, capable of responding but response may be inappropriate	5
Semi-comatose, responsive to visual stimuli	4
Semi-comatose, responsive to auditory stimuli	3
Semi-comatose, responsive only to repeated noxious stimuli	2
Comatose, unresponsive to repeated noxious stimuli	1

This provides a score of 3 to 18. The higher the score the better the prognosis.

Mouse biological data [11]

Lifespan (years)	1–2.5
Adult bodyweight (g)	Males: 20–40 Females: 20–60
Dentition	2 [I1/1 C0/0 P0/0 M3/3] Only incisors open-rooted
Number of digits	Front: 4 Rear: 5
Rectal temperature (°C)	~37.5
Heart rate (beats/min)	420–700
Respiratory rate (breaths/min)	100–250
Environmental temperature (°C)	24–25
Relative humidity (%)	45–55
Daily water intake	15 ml/100 g
Fluid therapy	100 ml/kg/24h
Diet	Omnivorous
Food intake per day per animal (g)	3–5
Coprophagy/Caecotrophy?	Yes
Oestrous type	Continuous polyoestrous
Post-partum oestrus?	Yes
Age at puberty (months)	1.5
Gestation length (days)	19–21
Oestrous cycle (days)	4–5
Oestrus duration (hours)	9–20
Litter size	7–12
Birth weight (g)	1–1.5
Altricial/Precocial	Altricial
Eyes open (days)	12–14
Age at weaning (days)	18–21

Number of pairs of teats	5
Minimum breeding age (months)	2
Ratio for breeding (M:F)	1:1–6 If polygamous remove female before parturition
Comments	They will eat the litter if disturbed in the first 2–3 days

Moxidectin [25, 26]
(Advocate, Cydectin, Endectrid, Multi-parasite, Prinovox)
POM-V
Formulations:
- Topical: 10 mg/ml, 25 mg/ml moxidectin with
  imidacloprid in spot-on pipette.
- Injectable: 1% solution.

DOSES

Dogs:
- Parasites (many): 2.5 mg/kg moxidectin. Apply once
  every month. Minimum dose recommendation 0.1 ml/kg.
- Demodicosis (severe): apply product weekly.

Cats: Parasites (many): 1.0 mg/kg moxidectin Apply once
every month. Minimum dose recommendation 0.1 ml/kg.

Mammals:
- Ferrets: 0.4 ml pipette monthly. If under heavy flea
  pressure can repeat once after 2 weeks
- Rabbits: 0.2–0.3 mg/kg p.o., repeat in 10 days
- Rodents: GI nematodes: 1 mg/kg of 2.5% v/w solution
  once.

Birds: 0.2 mg/kg topically prn.

Reptiles: Bearded dragons, Frillneck lizards: 0.2 ml/kg
topically q14d for 3 treatments.

Amphibians: 200 µg (micrograms)/kg s.c. q4months for
nematodes.

Fish: No information available.

NOTES

Neck pain — clinical approach [15]

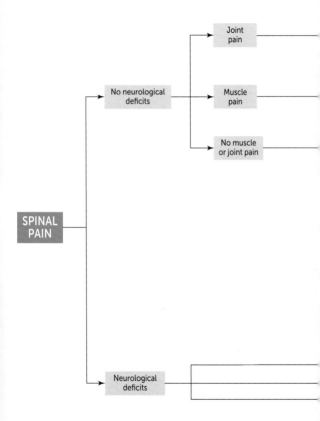

ANA = anti-nuclear antibody; CK = creatine kinase; CSF = cerebrospinal fluid; LE = lupus erythematosus; RhF = rheumatoid factor.

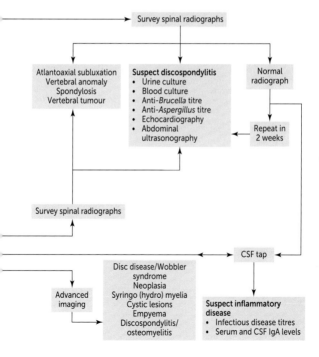

Suspect polyarthritis
- Joint tap analysis and culture
- Radiograph joints
- Antibody titres for infectious disease

- Blood and urine culture
- Serum LE, ANA, RhF
- Joint capsule biopsy
- Echocardiography
- Rule out intestinal disease
- Rule out systemic cancer

Suspect polymyositis
- Serum CK levels
- Electrophysiology
- Muscle biopsy

- Antibody titres for infectious disease
- Serum LE, ANA, RhF

Survey spinal radiographs

Atlantoaxial subluxation
Vertebral anomaly
Spondylosis
Vertebral tumour

Suspect discospondylitis
- Urine culture
- Blood culture
- Anti-*Brucella* titre
- Anti-*Aspergillus* titre
- Echocardiography
- Abdominal ultrasonography

Normal radiograph

Repeat in 2 weeks

Survey spinal radiographs

CSF tap

Advanced imaging

Disc disease/Wobbler syndrome
Neoplasia
Syringo (hydro) myelia
Cystic lesions
Empyema
Discospondylitis/osteomyelitis

Suspect inflammatory disease
- Infectious disease titres
- Serum and CSF IgA levels

Neurological examination [15]

Chief complaint

Historical background
Onset
Duration
Evolution   Static/Progressive/Regressive
                  Wax and wane/Episodic
Lateralization of signs
Animal background
Previous medical problems
Previous surgical problems
Previous travel
Vaccination status
Diet
Family history
Treatment

Neurological findings
Neurological exam   Normal/Abnormal
Abnormalities   Neurolocalization
-
-
-
-
-

Is the lesion?:   Focal   Multifocal   Diffuse
               Symmetrical Asymmetrical

Anatomical diagnosis Focal   Multifocal   Diffuse

☐ Forebrain   ☐ L4–L6
☐ Brainstem   ☐ L6–S3
☐ Cerebellar   ☐ Neuromuscular
☐ Vestibular: peripheral/central   ☐ Mononeuropathy
☐ C1–C5   ☐ Polyneuropathy
☐ C6–T2   ☐ Junctionopathy
☐ T3–L3   ☐ Myopathy

Comprehensive neurological examination form.
Cranial nerves: H = horizontal; L = large; M = mid-range; R = rotary;
S = small; V = vertical.

Suspected aetiological diagnosis

- ☐ Degenerative
- ☐ Anomalous
- ☐ Metabolic
- ☐ Neoplastic
- ☐ Nutritional
- ☐ Inflammatory/infectious
- ☐ Idiopathic
- ☐ Trauma
- ☐ Toxic
- ☐ Vascular

Recommended diagnostic tests:

Observation

Mental status	Normal/Abnormal
	Confusion/Depressed/Stuporous/Comatose
Behaviour	Normal/Abnormal
Body posture	Normal/Abnormal
	Head tilt/Head turn/Spinal curvature/
	Wide-based stance/Decerebrate/Decerebellate
	Schiff-Sherrington
Gait	Normal/Abnormal
Ataxia	Symmetrical/Asymmetrical
	Thoracic/Pelvic limbs
Paresis/plegia	Tetra/Para/Mono/Hemi
Circling	Left/Right
Lameness	

Involuntary movement

Postural reactions

Left	Right
Proprioceptive positioning	
Thoracic	
Pelvic	
Hopping	
Thoracic	
Pelvic	
Wheelbarrowing	
Extensor postural thrust	
Visual placing	
Tactile placing	

Comprehensive neurological examination form.
Cranial nerves: H = horizontal; L = large; M = mid-range; R = rotary;
S = small; V = vertical.

⟶

Cranial nerves

	Left		Right
		Facial symmetry	
		Palpebral (V + VII)	
		Corneal (V + VI, VII)	
		Oculovestibular (VIII + III, IV, VI)	
		Jaw tone (V)	
		Gag reflex (IX, X)	
		Tongue (XII)	
		Menace (Retina, II, forebrain + cerebellum, VII)	
		Nasal stimulation (V, forebrain)	
		Pupil size (Retina, II + III)	
	S M L	In light	S M L
	S M L	In dark (Sympathetic)	S M L
		Pupillary light reflex (Retina, II + III) Left eye Right eye	
		Nystagmus	
	H V R	Spontaneous (VIII)	H V R
	H V R	Positional	H V R
		Strabismus Permanent (III or IV or VI) Positional (VIII)	

Comprehensive neurological examination form.
Cranial nerves: H = horizontal; L = large; M = mid-range; R = rotary;
S = small; V = vertical.

Spinal reflexes

	Left	Right
Withdrawal thoracic (C6–T2)		
Extensor carpi radialis (C7–T2)		
Withdrawal pelvic (L6–S2)		
Patellar (L4–L6)		
Gastrocnemius (L6–S1)		
Perineal (S1–S3)		
Tail movement? Y/N		

Urinary function

Evidence of voluntary urination?	Y/N
Bladder distended?	Y/N
Easy bladder expression?	Y/N

Sensory evaluation

	Left	Right
Nociception		
Thoracic		
Pelvic		
Perineal		
Cutaneous trunci reflex		
Cutaneous sensation		
Thoracic		
Pelvic		
Specific nerve affected?		

Palpation/manipulation

Spinal pain?	Cervical/Thoracic/Lumbar/Sacral
Joint pain?	Y/N
Muscle pain?	Y/N
Neck movement	Normal/Abnormal

Comprehensive neurological examination form.
Cranial nerves: H = horizontal; L = large; M = mid-range; R = rotary;
S = small; V = vertical.

Non-steroidal anti-inflammatory drug (NSAID) poisoning **(URGENT)** [1]

Also known as: Aceclofenac, acemetacin, carprofen, celecoxib, dexibuprofen, dexketoprofen, diclofenac, etodolac, etoricoxib, fenbufen, flurbiprofen, ibuprofen, indometacin, ketoprofen, ketorolac, mavacoxib, meloxicam, nabumetone, naproxen, parecoxib, piroxicam, robenacoxib, sulindac, tiaprofenic acid, tolfenamic acid

Description/exposure

Non-steroidal anti-inflammatory drugs (NSAIDs) are common human (e.g. ibuprofen, naproxen, aspirin) and veterinary (e.g. carprofen, meloxicam, firocoxib) analgesics. Exposure may be accidental (especially with palatable chewable forms of the drugs) or by owner-induced overdose.

Mechanism of action

NSAIDs are competitive inhibitors of cyclo-oxygenase (COX) enzymes, resulting in decreased production of constitutive prostaglandins that are vital for homeostasis and maintenance of renal blood flow and gastric mucosal integrity. As such, toxicosis can result in gastrointestinal upset, including ulceration and acute kidney injury (AKI). In dogs, ibuprofen doses >100—125 mg/kg can result in gastric ulceration, doses >175—200 mg/kg can result in AKI and doses >400 mg/kg are associated with seizures and death. For veterinary NSAIDs in dogs, the general guideline is that >5 times the therapeutic dose may result in gastrointestinal signs, whilst >10 times the therapeutic dose may result in AKI. Cats are considered to be at least twice as sensitive to NSAIDs as dogs.

Clinical presentation

Clinical signs of NSAID toxicosis may include anorexia, vomiting, haematemesis, diarrhoea, melena, pallor, acute abdomen, uraemic halitosis, polyuria, polydipsia, anuria and colic.

Diagnostics

A minimum database of haematology, serum biochemistry and urinalysis (including urine specific gravity prior to fluid therapy) is recommended. Monitoring for clinicopathological evidence of gastrointestinal ulceration (e.g. hypoproteinaemia, anaemia and elevated blood urea nitrogen), perforation (e.g. initial hyperglycaemia, hypoglycaemia, presence of band neutrophils, cytological evidence of septic peritoneal effusion) or AKI (e.g. hyperphosphataemia, renal azotaemia, isosthenuria prior to fluid administration) should be performed.

Treatment

Depending on the toxic dose ingested, aggressive treatment of NSAID exposure is recommended. Induction of emesis and administration of activated charcoal are often recommended. Multiple doses of activated charcoal should be considered if the NSAID undergoes enterohepatic recirculation (e.g. carprofen and ibuprofen) or has a long half-life (e.g. naproxen has a half-life of 72 hours). Gastrointestinal medications should include antiemetics and ulcer prophylaxis with antacids (e.g. H2 blockers or proton pump inhibitors) and sucralfate. Synthetic prostaglandins (e.g. misoprostol) can be considered to increase gastric mucus production, mucosal blood flow and healing. However, misprostol has unknown efficacy in the prevention or treatment of gastric ulcers. Aggressive intravenous fluid therapy is recommended to maintain renal perfusion and to aid in vasodilation of the renal vessels.

Prognosis

With aggressive treatment, the prognosis for NSAID toxicosis is excellent, if treated early. However, once azotaemia, oliguria or anuria has developed, the prognosis is poor to guarded.

NOTES

Oclacitinib [25]
(Apoquel) POM-V

Formulations: Oral: 3.6 mg, 5.4 mg, 16 mg tablets.

DOSES

Dogs, Cats: Atopic dermatitis: 0.4–0.6 mg/kg p.o. q12h for 14 days, then q24h for maintenance.

Apoquel (from datasheet)				
Dose rate	Patient bodyweight (kg)	No. of tablets per dose, twice daily (initial dose) followed by once daily (maintenance dose)		
		3.6 mg	**5.4 mg**	**16 mg**
Dogs				
0.4–0.6 mg/kg	3.0–4.4	½		
	4.5–5.9		½	
	6.0–8.9	1		
	9.0–13.4		1	
	13.5–19.9			½
	20.0–26.9		2	
	27.0–39.9			1
	40.0–54.9			1½
	55.0–80.0			2

NOTES

Oesophagostomy tube placement [4]

EQUIPMENT

- Oesophagostomy tube (red rubber tube, standard polyurethane feeding tube or silicone feeding tube):
  - Cats: 10–14 Fr; 23 cm long
  - Dogs: 14–24 Fr; 40 cm long
- Long curved forceps, e.g. Rochester–Carmalt
- No. 15 or 20 scalpel blade and holder
- 25 mm wide adhesive tape
- Non-absorbable suture material, needle and needle-holders
- Sterile dressing to cover the tube site
- Light bandage for the neck
- Cotton wool or soft swabs
- 4% chlorhexidine gluconate or 10% povidone–iodine
- 70% surgical spirit
- 1 sterile fenestrated skin drape

TECHNIQUE

1. Insert the curved forceps through the mouth and into the oesophagus, to the mid-cervical region.
2. Turn the tip of the forceps laterally and use the scalpel to make a 5–10 mm skin incision over the point of the tips.

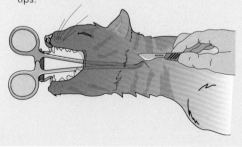

TECHNIQUE *continued*

3. Bluntly dissect through the subcutaneous tissues and make an incision into the oesophagus over the tips of the forceps.
4. Push the tips of the forceps outwards through the incision to the external surface.
5. Measure the oesophagostomy tube from this point to the 7th intercostal space (distal oesophagus) and mark the tube with a piece of adhesive tape.
6. Open the tips of the forceps and grasp the distal end of the feeding tube.

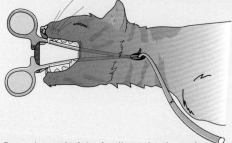

7. Draw the end of the feeding tube through the oesophagostomy incision and rostrally into the pharynx to exit the mouth.

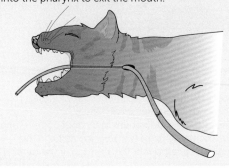

TECHNIQUE *continued*

8. Disengage the tips of the forceps, curl the tip of the tube back into the mouth and feed it into the oesophagus.

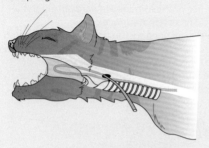

9. Visually inspect the oropharynx to confirm that the tube is no longer present in the oropharynx.
10. The tube should slide easily back and forth a few centimetres, confirming that it has straightened.

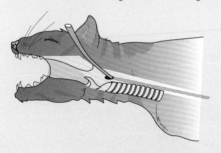

11. Secure the tube by placement of a "Chinese finger-trap"/"Roman Sandal" suture.
12. Take a thoracic radiograph to confirm correct tube placement: the tip of the tube should be in the distal oesophagus, not the stomach. If the tube has

an integral radiodense marker, iodinated (not barium) contrast medium can be instilled into the tube to aid visualization.

13. Cover the tube site with a sterile dressing and place a soft padded loose neck bandage.

NOTES

Omeprazole [25, 26]

(Gastrogard, Losec*, Mepradec*, Zanprol*) POM-V, POM

Formulations:

- Oral: 10 mg, 20 mg, 40 mg capsules, gastro-resistant tablets, MUPS (multiple unit pellet system) tablets.
- Injectable: 40 mg vial for reconstitution for i.v. injection. Powder for solution for infusion must only be dissolved in either 100 ml of 0.9% NaCl or 5% dextrose. Powder should be initially dissolved in 5 ml of liquid to dissolve the powder then immediately diluted to 100 ml. Do not use if any particles are present in the reconstituted solution. Once reconstituted, the solution should be used within 12 hours (in 0.9% saline) or 6 hours (in 5% glucose).

DOSES

Dogs: 0.5–1.5 mg/kg i.v., p.o. q12–24h for a maximum of 8 weeks.

Cats: 0.75–1 mg/kg p.o. q24h for a maximum of 8 weeks.

Mammals:
- Primates: 0.4 mg/kg p.o. q12h
- Ferrets: 0.7–4 mg/kg p.o. q24h for a maximum of 8 weeks.

Birds, Reptiles, Amphibians, Fish: No information available.

Ortolani test [5]

Indications/Use

- To detect hip laxity in the young dog (to support a diagnosis of hip dysplasia).

NOTE

Not all dogs with hip dysplasia show a positive Ortolani sign. For example, dogs with gross subluxation or luxation of the femoral head, and dogs in which capsular fibrosis has stabilized the hip joint will not show the sign.

Patient preparation and positioning

- May be attempted in the conscious animal but is potentially painful and therefore best performed with the dog heavily sedated or under general anaesthesia.
- The animal may be positioned in lateral or dorsal recumbency. The description below applies to lateral recumbency.

Technique

1. Position the stifle in mild flexion and grasp it with one hand, with the other hand placed on the dorsal aspect of the pelvis to stabilize it.
2. Apply firm pressure to the stifle in a dorsal direction in an attempt to subluxate the hip joint.
3. Whilst maintaining dorsal pressure on the stifle, gently abduct the limb until a 'click' or 'clunk' is detected.
   - If the dorsal acetabular rim is intact, the femoral head falls abruptly into the acetabulum.
   - In dogs with a poor dorsal acetabular rim, the femoral head appears to slide back into the acetabulum.

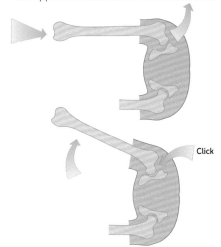

4. Whilst maintaining dorsal pressure on the stifle, if the limb is now adducted, re-luxation of the hip will occur.

Results

■ The 'click' or 'clunk' (see Step 3) represents the relocation of the femoral head within the acetabulum. This is the positive Ortolani sign, consistent with hip joint laxity.

NOTES

Otitis externa/media – clinical approach [11]

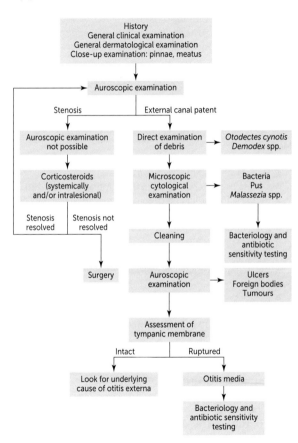

A practical approach to otitis externa and otitis media. (Adapted from DN Carlotti)

Oxytetracycline [25, 26]

(Aquatet [Pharmaq], Engemycin, Oxycare) POM-V

Formulations:

- Injectable: 100 mg/ml solution.
- Oral: 50 mg, 100 mg, 250 mg tablets. Feed supplement and soluble powders also available.

DOSES

Dogs: 10 mg/kg i.m., s.c. q24h; 50 mg/kg loading dose, then 25 mg/kg p.o. q12h for up to 5 days. Give oral dose on an empty stomach.

Cats: 10 mg/kg i.m., s.c. q24h.

Mammals:

- Primates: 10 mg/kg s.c., i.m. q24h
- Hedgehogs: 50 mg/kg p.o. q12h
- Ferrets, Hamsters, Gerbils: 20–25 mg/kg i.m. q8–12h
- Rabbits: 15 mg/kg i.m. q12h or 30 mg/kg of the 5–10% non-depot preparation s.c. q72h
- Chinchillas: 15 mg/kg i.m. q12h or 50 mg/kg p.o. q12h
- Guinea pigs: 5 mg/kg i.m. q12h
- Rats: 20 mg/kg i.m. q8–12h or 10–20 mg/kg p.o. q8h
- Mice: 100 mg/kg s.c. q12h or 10–20 mg/kg p.o. q8h.

Birds:

- Raptors: 25–50 mg/kg p.o. q8h
- Parrots: 50–100 mg/kg s.c. q2–3d (long-acting preparation)
- Passerines: 100 mg/kg p.o. q24h or 4–12 mg/l water for 7 days
- Pigeons: 50 mg/kg p.o. q6h or 80 mg/kg i.m. q48h (long-acting preparation) or 130–400 mg/l water.

Reptiles: 6–10 mg/kg p.o., i.m., i.v. q24h.

Amphibians: 25–50 mg/kg p.o., s.c., i.m. q24h or 100 mg/l for a 1 hour bath.

Fish: 10–100 mg/l (freshwater fish) by prolonged immersion for 1–3 days, if poor response then change 50% of the water and repeat, or 55–83 mg/kg p.o. q24h for 10 days or 10–50 mg/kg i.m., i.p. q24h for 5–10 days.

Oxytocin [25, 26]
(Oxytocin S) POM-V

Formulations: Injectable: 10 IU/ml solution.

DOSES

Dogs:
- Obstetric indications: 0.1–0.5 IU/kg i.m., s.c. q30min for up to 3 doses.
- Milk let-down: 2–20 IU/dog i.m., s.c. once.

Cats:
- Obstetric indications: 0.1–0.5 IU/kg i.m., s.c. q30min for up to 2 doses.
- Milk let-down: 1–10 IU/cat i.m., s.c. once.

Mammals:
- Primates: 5–20 IU/animal i.v., i.m.
- Ferrets: 0.2–3.0 IU/kg s.c., i.m.
- Rabbits: 0.1–3.0 IU/kg s.c., i.m.
- Rodents: 0.2–3.0 IU/kg s.c., i.m., i.v.
- Mice: (milk let-down) 6.25 IU/kg s.c.

Birds: Do not use.

Reptiles: Egg retention: 2–10 IU/kg i.m. q90min for a maximum of 3 doses. Better effect if calcium therapy used first.
- Red-eared sliders: 2 IU/kg i.m., i.v.

Amphibians, Fish: No information available.

NOTES

NOTES

NOTES

Pain scoring – cat [7]

Pain score	Example	Psychological and behavioural	Response to palpation	Body tension
0		☐ Animal is sleeping and cannot be evaluated		
		☐ Content and quiet when unattended ☐ Comfortable when resting ☐ Interested in or curious about surroundings	☐ Not bothered by palpation of wound or surgery site, or to palpation elsewhere	Minimal
1		☐ Signs are often subtle and not easily detected in the hospital setting; more likely to be detected by the owner(s) at home ☐ Earliest signs at home may be withdrawal from surroundings or change in normal routine ☐ In the hospital, may be content or slightly unsettled ☐ Less interested in surroundings but will look around to see what is going on	☐ May or may not react to palpation of wound or surgery site	Mild
2		☐ Decreased responsiveness, seeks solitude ☐ Quiet, loss of brightness in eyes ☐ Lays curled up or sits tucked up (all four feet under body, shoulders hunched, head held slightly lower than shoulders, tail curled tightly around body) with eyes partially or mostly closed ☐ Hair coat appears rough or fluffed ☐ May intensively groom an area that is painful or irritating ☐ Decreased appetite, not interested in food	☐ Responds aggressively or tries to escape if painful area is palpated or approached ☐ Tolerates attention, may even perk up when petted as long as painful area is avoided	Mild to moderate **Reassess analgesic plan**

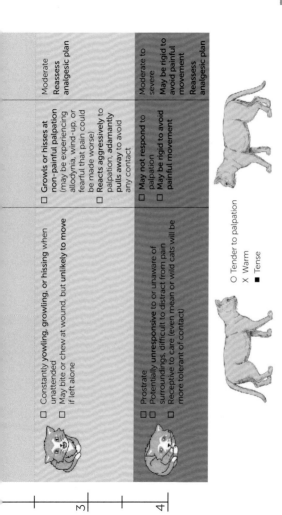

		Moderate Reassess analgesic plan
☐ Constantly yowling, growling, or hissing when unattended ☐ May bite or chew at wound, but unlikely to move if left alone	☐ Growls or hisses at non-painful palpation (may be experiencing allodynia, wind-up, or fearful that pain could be made worse) ☐ Reacts aggressively to palpation, adamantly pulls away to avoid any contact	
☐ Prostrate ☐ Potentially unresponsive to or unaware of surroundings, difficult to distract from pain ☐ Receptive to care (even mean or wild cats will be more tolerant of contact)	☐ May not respond to palpation ☐ May be rigid to avoid painful movement	Moderate to severe May be rigid to avoid painful movement Reassess analgesic plan

3

4

O Tender to palpation
X Warm
■ Tense

The Colorado Feline Acute Pain Scale. (Reproduced with permission from Peter W. Hellyer, College of Veterinary Medicine and Biomedical Sciences, Colorado State University, USA)

Pain scoring – dog [7]

Dog's name .... Date / / Time ....

Hospital number ....

Procedure or condition..

....

In the sections below please circle the appropriate score in each list and sum these to give the total score

A. Look at dog in kennel

Is the dog

(i)		(ii)	
Quiet	0	Ignoring any wound or painful area	0
Crying or whimpering	1	Looking at wound or painful area	1
Groaning	2	Licking wound or painful area	2
Screaming	3	Rubbing wound or painful area	3
		Chewing wound or painful area	4

In the case of spinal, pelvic or multiple limb fractures, or where assistance is required to aid locomotion, do not carry out section **B** and proceed to **C**. Please tick if this is the case ☐ then proceed to **C**

B. Put lead on dog and lead out of the kennel

When the dog rises/walks is it?

(iii)

Normal	0
Lame	1
Slow or reluctant	2
Stiff	3
It refuses to move	4

C. If it has a wound or painful area including abdomen, apply gentle pressure 2 inches round the site

Does it? (iv)

Do nothing	0
Look round	1
Flinch	2
Growl or guard area	3
Snap	4
Cry	5

D. Overall

Is the dog? (v)

Happy and content or happy and bouncy	0
Quiet	1
Indifferent or non-responsive to surroundings	2
Nervous or anxious or fearful	3
Depressed or non-responsive to stimulation	4

Is the dog? (vi)

Comfortable	0
Unsettled	1
Restless	2
Hunched or tense	3
Rigid	4

Total score (i+ii+iii+iv+v+vi) = ...

The Glasgow Composite Measure Pain Score (short form).
(© University of Glasgow 2008)

Guidance for use of the CMPS-SF

The short form composite measure pain score (CMPS-SF) can be applied quickly and reliably in a clinical setting and has been designed as a clinical decision making tool which was developed for dogs in acute pain. It includes 30 descriptor options within 6 behavioural categories, including mobility. Within each category, the descriptors are ranked numerically according to their associated pain severity and the person carrying out the assessment chooses the descriptor within each category which best fits the dog's behaviour/condition. It is important to carry out the assessment procedure as described on the questionnaire, following the protocol closely. The pain score is the sum of the rank scores. The maximum score for the 6 categories is 24, or 20 if mobility is impossible to assess. The total CMPS-SF score has been shown to be a useful indicator of analgesic requirement and the recommended analgesic intervention level is 6/24 or 5/20.

NOTES

Paracetamol (Acetaminophen) [25, 26]

(Paracetamol, Pardale V (paracetamol and codeine phosphate), Perfalgan) P, POM, POM-V

Formulations:

- Oral: 500 mg tablet; 120 mg/5 ml, 250 mg/5 ml suspensions; 400 mg paracetamol and 9 mg codeine phosphate tablet (Pardale V)
- Injectable: 10 mg/ml solution.

DOSES

Dogs: 10 mg/kg p.o., i.v. q12h. Dose of the Pardale V preparation is 1 tablet per 12 kg bodyweight.

Pardale V (from datasheet)	
Bodyweight (kg)	**No. of tablets per dose, three times daily for a maximum of 5 days**
Dogs	
<6	½
6–18	½–1½
18–42	1½–3½

Cats: Do not use.

Mammals:
- Primates: 5–10 mg/kg p.o. q6h
- Rabbits: 200–500 mg/kg p.o.
- Rodents: 1–2 mg/ml of drinking water (use flavoured products).

Birds, Reptiles, Amphibians, Fish: No information available.

NOTES

Paracetamol poisoning (CAUTION)[1]

Also known as: Acetaminophen

Description/exposure

Paracetamol (*N*-acetyl-*p*-aminophenol), otherwise known as acetaminophen (APAP), is an over-the-counter (OTC) analgesic and antipyretic for humans. There are authorized products for use in dogs that are a combination of paracetamol and codeine. Most animals are exposed through accidental ingestion or uninformed owner administration.

Mechanism of action

Normally paracetamol is metabolized into a non-toxic conjugate. Toxicosis occurs when glucuronidation and sulfation pathways are saturated, in which case a toxic metabolite *N*-acetyl-para-benzoquinoneimine (NAPQI) is generated via the cytochrome p450 pathway. NAPQI can be conjugated with glutathione and detoxified, but NAPQI accumulation results in oxidative injury, methaemoglobinaemia (metHb) and hepatic injury. Cats have a decreased capacity for glucuronidation, are more susceptible to toxicosis and have a much lower toxic dose (10 mg/kg) compared with dogs (100–150 mg/kg).

Clinical presentation

Cats may present with severe, acute clinical signs within an hour of exposure. Swelling of the face and paws, gastrointestinal signs (e.g. anorexia, hypersalivation and vomiting), respiratory distress, brown mucus membranes, cyanosis, tachypnoea and dyspnoea may be seen. In dogs, the clinical signs may be similar, although hepatic failure is more likely to be seen than the development of metHb. Signs of hepatic failure may take 24–48 hours to manifest and include malaise, anorexia, vomiting, hypersalivation, elevated liver enzymes, icterus, hepatic encephalopathy and death. Rarely, keratoconjunctivitis sicca has been reported in dogs secondary to paracetamol exposure, even at sub-toxic levels.

⟶

Diagnostics

Haematology, serum biochemistry and a blood smear should be performed. A haematocrit tube should be evaluated for the presence of metHb (the blood will be a chocolate brown colour). While not commonly available, a multi-wavelength co-oximeter can be used to measure metHb. Human hospitals may be able to measure quantitative paracetamol levels, which can help establish the prognosis and determine whether treatment is necessary.

Treatment

As paracetamol is rapidly absorbed from the gastrointestinal tract (with peak plasma levels being achieved within as little as 20 minutes after ingestion), the induction of emesis is not warranted. Immediate use of activated charcoal with a cathartic is preferred. Stabilization is warranted in severely affected paracetamol toxicosis cases and includes oxygen therapy, intravenous fluid therapy, antiemetic medication, blood products (to provide functional haemoglobin) and supportive care. Antioxidants (e.g. vitamin C) and hepatoprotectants or glutathione precursors (SAMe and NAC) reduce and limit the production of NAPQI, the harmful metabolite, and should be instituted immediately. The use of cimetidine (to inhibit cytochrome p450 metabolism) is no longer recommended for paracetamol toxicosis, as it has not been found to be beneficial. In cases with severe metHb, the use of methylene blue can be considered; its use should be limited to dogs due to the risk of Heinz body anaemia when used in cats. Supportive therapy for liver injury or failure may be indicated. In dogs, if liver enzymes are within normal limits after 48 hours of NAC treatment, the patient can be successfully discharged. The veterinary surgeon is referred to an appropriate reference book for further information on how to treat hepatic failure.

Prognosis

Poor in patients with severe hepatoxicity.

Patellar luxations – grading [13]

Grade I

The patella can be manually luxated but returns to a normal position when released.

Grade II

The patella may luxate during stifle flexion or manual manipulation and remains luxated until stifle extension or manual replacement occurs. This grade covers a broad spectrum of disease severity in that the patella may luxate infrequently or frequently.

Grade III

The patella is permanently luxated but can be manually replaced. It reluxates spontaneously when manual pressure is removed.

Grade IV

The patella is permanently luxated and cannot be replaced.

Percentage solutions conversion table [25]

The concentration of a solution may be expressed on the basis of weight per unit volume (w/v) or volume per unit volume (v/v).

% w/v = number of grams of a substance in 100 ml of a liquid

% v/v = number of ml of a substance in 100 ml of liquid

% Solution	g or ml/100 ml	mg/ml	Solution strength
100	100	1000	1:1
10	10	100	1:10
1	1	10	1:100
0.1	0.1	1	1:1000
0.01	0.01	0.1	1:10,000

Pericardial effusion key points [12]

- Typical clinical signs/physical examination findings: weakness, syncope, distended jugular veins, weak femoral pulses, tachycardia, muffled heart sounds and ascites. Patients with acute cardiac tamponade may present in cardiogenic shock.
- Diagnosis: echocardiography is the most sensitive and specific test for diagnosing and assessing the clinical relevance of a pericardial effusion.
- Treatment: pericardiocentesis is the treatment of choice for pericardial decompression and should be performed as an emergency procedure whenever there is evidence of cardiac tamponade (RA or RV collapse identified on echocardiography). In cats, pericardiocentesis is generally not necessary because cardiac tamponade is rare.
- Prognosis: The prognosis for dogs with pericardial effusion is quite variable; it may be good to excellent in cases of idiopathic pericarditis, fair in cases of heart base tumours (chemodectomas) or mesotheliomas, and poor in cases of haemangiosarcoma. In cats with pericardial effusion secondary to CHF and advanced cardiac disease, the prognosis is typically poor.

NOTES

Pimobendan [25, 26]

(Cardisure, Fortekor-Plus, Pimocard, Vetmedin) POM-V

Formulations:

- Injectable: 0.75 mg/ml solution (5 ml, 10 ml vials).
- Oral: 1.25 mg, 5 mg hard capsules or 1.25 mg, 2.5 mg, 5 mg, 10 mg chewable tablets (Vetmedin); 1.25 mg, 2.5 mg, 5 mg, 10 mg flavoured tablets (Cardisure, Pimocard). Also available in compound preparation with pimobendan (Fortekor Plus) in the following formulations, 1.25 mg pimobendan/2.5 mg benazepril, 5 mg pimobendan/10 mg benazepril.

DOSES

Dogs: 0.15 mg/kg i.v. single dose. Oral pimobendan can be continued 12 hours after administration of the injection.

Dogs, Cats: 0.1–0.3 mg/kg p.o. q12h one hour before food.

Vetmedin (from datasheet)				
Dose rate	Patient bodyweight (kg)	Daily dosage (mg)	No. of tablets required, twice daily	
			1.25 mg	*5.0 mg*
Dogs				
0.2–0.6 mg/kg	<5	1.25	½	
	5–10	2.5	1	
	11–20	5		½
	21–40	10		1
	41–60	20		2
	>60	30		3

Mammals:

- Sugar gliders: 0.3–0.5 mg/kg p.o. q12h
- Hedgehogs: 0.3 mg/kg p.o. q12h
- Ferrets: 0.5 mg/kg p.o. q12h
- Rabbits: 0.1–0.3 mg/kg p.o. q12–24h
- Rodents: 0.2–0.4 mg/kg p.o. q12h.

Birds: 0.25 mg/kg p.o. q12h.

Reptiles, Amphibians, Fish: No information available.

Polyuria and polydipsia – diagnostic approach [14]

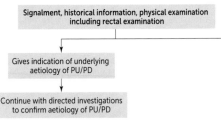

Signalment, historical information, physical examination including rectal examination

⬇

Gives indication of underlying aetiology of PU/PD

⬇

Continue with directed investigations to confirm aetiology of PU/PD

⬇

Provides likely diagnosis/aetiology for PU/PD
- Azotaemia
  - Differentiate pre-renal, renal, post-renal azotaemia
  - Differentiate acute kidney injury *versus* chronic kidney disease
  - Consider hypoadrenocorticoid crisis in the acute patient
- Hypercalcaemia
  - Document persistence
  - Confirm ionized hypercalcaemia
  - Investigate underlying aetiology of hypercalcaemia
- Diabetes mellitus
  - Consider assessment of fructosamine
  - In a cat consider the possibility of hypersomatotropism (acromegaly)
- Renal glucosuria
  - Differentiate primary renal glucosuria from complex tubulopathy
  - Evaluate for potential underlying aetiology of glucosuria (e.g. drugs, toxins, hepatic disease, 'jerky' treats)
- Hypokalaemia
  - Investigate underlying aetiology of hypokalaemia
- Hyperthyroidism
  - Initiate treatment and monitor for unmasking of chronic kidney disease

ACTH = adrenocorticotropic hormone; GFR = glomerular filtration rate; PD = polydipsia; PU = polyuria; SDMA = symmetric dimethylarginine. For further information see the *BSAVA Manual of Canine and Feline Nephrology and Urology, 3rd edition.*

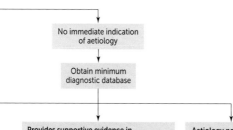

No immediate indication
of aetiology

Obtain minimum
diagnostic database

**Provides supportive evidence in
conjunction with clinical assessment for:**
- Pyelonephritis
- Hyperadrenocorticism
- Hypoadrenocorticism
- Hepatic disease
- Non-azotaemic kidney disease

Proceed with additional diagnostic
investigation to confirm suspected diagnosis

Aetiology not identified
Continue with advanced
diagnostic investigation

Confirmation of diagnosis:
- **Pyelonephritis**
  - Abdominal/renal ultrasonography/computed tomography
  - Repeat urine culture
  - Pyelocentesis for culture
- **Hyperadrenocorticism**
  - ACTH stimulation test
  - Low dose dexamethasone suppression test
  - Diagnostic imaging of adrenal glands/pituitary
- **Hypoadrenocorticism**
  - ACTH stimulation test
- **Hepatic disease/hepatic failure/portovascular anomaly**
  - Bile acid stimulation test
  - Ammonia concentration
  - Abdominal ultrasonography/radiography/computed tomography angiography
  - Urine sediment examination (urate crystalluria)
  - Hepatic fine-needle aspiration/biopsy
- **Non-azotaemic kidney disease**
  - Serial assessment of urine specific gravity
  - Diagnostic imaging of kidney (ultrasound examination, computed tomography)
  - Measurement of serum SDMA
  - GFR measurement (plasma iohexol clearance)

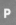

Potassium salts (Potassium chloride, Potassium gluconate) [25]

(Kaminox, Tumil-K) general sale

Formulations:

- Injectable: 20% KCl solution (2 g KCl/10 ml; 26 mmol K+). Before use dilute the solution with at least 70 times its volume of sodium chloride intravenous fluid.
- Oral: Tablets containing 2 mEq potassium gluconate; Powder (2 mEq per ¼ teaspoon) (Tumil-K); Liquid 1 mEq/ml potassium gluconate formulated with a range of amino acids, B vitamins and iron (Kaminox). Note: 1 mmol/l = 1 mEq/l.

Serum potassium	Amount to be added to 250 ml 0.9% NaCl
<2 mmol/l	20 mmol
2–2.5 mmol/l	15 mmol
2.5–3 mmol/l	10 mmol
3–3.5 mmol/l	7 mmol
3.5–5.5 mmol/l	5 mmol (minimum daily need in anorectic patients)

DOSES

Dogs: Correction of hypokalaemia: Intravenous doses must be titrated for each patient; dilute concentrated solutions prior to use (normally to 20–60 mmol/l). Rate of i.v. infusion should not exceed 0.5 mmol/kg/h, especially when concentration in replacement fluid is >60 mmol/l. Use of fluid pumps is recommended. Oral: Replacement dose needs to be titrated to effect to maintain mid-range normal values in each individual patient. Starting doses are 2 mEq per 4.5 kg in food q12h or 2.2 mEq per 100 kcal required energy intake.

Cats: Correction of hypokalaemia: Intravenous doses as for dogs. Oral: Replacement dose needs to be titrated to effect to maintain mid-range normal values in each individual patient. Starting doses are 2.2 mEq per 4.5 kg in food q12h or 2–6 mEq/cat/day p.o. in divided doses q8–12h.

Praziquantel [25, 26]

(Broadline, Cazitel, Cestem, Droncit, Droncit Spot-on, Drontal, Dolpac, Endoguard, Fluke-Solve, Milbactor, Milbemax, Milpro, Prazitel, Profender, Veloxa, various other authorized proprietary preparations) POM-V, NFA-VPS, AVM-GSL

Formulations:

- Oral: 10 mg, 20 mg, 25 mg, 30 mg, 40 mg, 50 mg, 125 mg, 144 mg, 150 mg, 175 mg tablets.
- Topical: 20 mg, 25 mg, 30 mg, 60 mg, 75 mg, 96 mg in spot-on pipettes.
- Immersion: 10 g, 100 g sachets (Fluke-Solve).

DOSES

Dogs: 5.0 mg/kg p.o. 8 mg/kg spot-on.

Cats: 5.0 mg/kg p.o; 8 mg/kg spot-on.

Drontal (from datasheet)		
Dose rate	Patient bodyweight (kg)	No. of tablets required
Dogs		
15 mg/kg bodyweight febantel, 14.4 mg/kg pyrantel and 5 mg/kg praziquantel	**Drontal Plus Flavour Tablets / Drontal Plus Flavour Bone Shaped Tablets**	
	3–5	½
	6–10	1
	11–15	1½
	16–20	2
	21–25	2½
	26–30	3
	31–35	3 ½
	36–40	4
	Drontal Plus XL Flavour Tablets	
	17.5	½
	>17.5–35	1
	>35–52.5	1½
	>52.5–70	2

Drontal (from datasheet)		
Dose rate	**Patient bodyweight (kg)**	**No. of tablets required**
Cats		
57.5 mg/kg bodyweight pyrantel embonate and 5 mg/kg praziquantel	*Drontal Cat Tablets*	
	2 kg	½
	4 kg	1
	6 kg	1½
	8 kg	2
	Drontal Cat XL Film-coated Tablets	
	6	1

Mammals:
- Primates: 20 mg/kg (cestodes) or 40 mg/kg (trematodes) p.o. once
- Hedgehogs: 7 mg/kg p.o., s.c., repeat in 14 days
- Ferrets: 5–10 mg/kg p.o., repeat in 10–14 days
- Rabbits: 5–10 mg/kg p.o., repeat in 10 days
- Gerbils, Rats, Mice: 30 mg/kg p.o. q14d (for 3 treatments).

Birds:
- Pigeons: 10–20 mg/kg p.o. or 7.5 mg/kg s.c., repeat in 10–14 days
- Other birds: 10 mg/kg i.m., repeat in 7–10 days.

Reptiles: 5–8 mg/kg p.o., repeat in 2 weeks in most species. Profender has been used topically at 1.12 ml/kg, corresponding to 24 mg emodepside and 96 mg praziquantel/kg, once.

Amphibians: 8–24 mg/kg p.o., s.c., intracoelomic q7–21d or 10 mg/l bath for 3 hours repeat q7–21d.

Fish: 2 mg/l by immersion, repeat every 3 weeks for 3 doses.

NOTES

Pre-anaesthetic drug combinations used in cats and dogs [7]

Drug combination		
Drug 1	*Drug 2*	
Acepromazine (0.01–0.05 mg/kg)	+ Buprenorphine (20 µg/kg) + Butorphanol (0.2–0.4 mg/kg) + Hydromorphone (0.05–0.15 mg/kg) + Methadone (0.2–0.5 mg/kg) + Morphine (0.2–0.5 mg/kg) + Pethidine (meperidine) (3–5 mg/kg)	
Dexmedetomidine (1–10 µg/kg) Use 1–3 µg/kg i.v. Doses up to 10 µg/kg may be used i.m. if profound sedation is required	+ Buprenorphine (20 µg/kg) + Butorphanol (0.2–0.4 mg/kg) + Hydromorphone (0.1 mg/kg) + Methadone (0.1–0.2 mg/kg) + Morphine (0.1–0.2 mg/kg) + Pethidine (3–5 mg/kg)	
Dexmedetomidine (1–10 µg/kg) Use 1–3 µg/kg i.v. Doses up to 10 µg/kg may be used i.m. if profound sedation is required	+ Diazepam (0.2–0.3 mg/kg) + Midazolam (0.2–0.3 mg/kg)	
Midazolam (0.3–0.4 mg/kg)	+ Butorphanol (0.2–0.4 mg/kg) + Hydromorphone (0.05–0.15 mg/kg) + Methadone (0.2–0.5 mg/kg) + Morphine (0.2–0.5 mg/kg) + Pethidine (3–5 mg/kg)	
Midazolam (0.2–0.3 mg/kg)	+ Ketamine (2–5 mg/kg)	

ASA = American Society of Anesthesiologists physical status classification; IPPV = intermittent positive pressure ventilation.

Route of administration	Species	Patient selection
i.m. or i.v. i.m. or i.v. i.m. or i.v. i.m. or i.v. i.m. i.m.	Cat and dog	ASA 1–3 patients, depending on assessment of cardiovascular function. Use lower dose of acepromazine in ASA 2–3 patients. Use lower dose range when drugs are given i.v.
i.m. or i.v. i.m. or i.v. i.m. or i.v. i.m. or i.v. i.m. i.m.	Cat and dog	ASA 1–2 patients For routine administration of these combinations cardiovascular function should be normal. Exceptions may be made in some circumstances. Use lower end of dose range when drugs are given i.v.
i.v. i.m. or i.v.	Dog	ASA 1–2 patients For routine administration of these combinations, cardiovascular function should be normal. Exceptions may be made in some circumstances. Useful for non-painful procedures such as diagnostic imaging. Use lower end of dose range when drugs are given i.v.
i.m. or i.v. i.m. or i.v. i.m. or i.v. i.m. i.m.	Dog, rarely cat	ASA 3–5 patients Provides good cardiovascular stability. Excitation may occur after i.v. administration; sedation is unreliable if given i.m. Avoid butorphanol if the animal is in pain. Use lower end of dose range when drugs are given i.v.
i.m. or i.v.	Cat	ASA 2–4 patients Avoid in patients with hypertrophic cardiomyopathy. Higher dose of ketamine may induce anaesthesia. Use lower end of dose range when drugs are given i.v.

Drug combination		
Drug 1	**Drug 2**	
Midazolam (0.3–0.4 mg/kg)	+ Fentanyl (2–5 µg/kg)	
Zolazepam + tiletamine	Available as a proprietary mixture (Telazol® or Zoletil®) Dose range for pre-anaesthetic medication 3–6 mg/kg	
Alfaxalone (1–3 mg/kg) Use lower dose range in combination with other drugs. Use higher dose s.c.	+ Methadone (0.2–0.5 mg/kg) + Buprenorphine (20 µg/kg) + Butorphanol (0.2–0.4 mg/kg)	
Morphine (0.2–0.5 mg/kg) Methadone (0.2–0.5 mg/kg) Hydromorphone (0.05–0.1 mg/kg)		

ASA = American Society of Anesthesiologists physical status classification; IPPV = intermittent positive pressure ventilation.

NOTES

Route of administration	Species	Patient selection
i.v.	Cat and dog	ASA 3–5 patients Provides good cardiovascular stability. Be prepared to induce anaesthesia to allow endotracheal intubation and IPPV if apnoea occurs. Use lower end of dose range when drugs are given i.v.
i.m. or i.v.	Cat and dog	As above for midazolam/ketamine mixture. Recovery can be stormy in dogs. Use lower end of dose range when drugs are given i.v.
i.m. or s.c. i.m. or s.c. i.m. or s.c.	Cat and dog	Volume limits utility in most dogs. Midazolam (0.2–0.3 mg/kg) may be added to this combination to provide increased sedation in anxious or fearful cats and dogs
i.m. i.m. or i.v. i.m. or i.v.	Cat and dog	ASA 4–5 patients or young animals. Use lower end of dose range when drugs are given i.v.

NOTES

Prednisolone [25, 26]

(PLT, Prednicare, Prednidale, Pred-forte*) POM-V

Formulations:

- Ophthalmic: Prednisolone acetate 0.5%, 1% suspensions in 5 ml, 10 ml bottles (Pred-forte).
- Topical: Prednisolone is a component of many topical dermatological, otic and ophthalmic preparations.
- Injectable: Prednisolone sodium succinate 10 mg/ml solution; 7.5 mg/ml suspension plus 2.5 mg/ml dexamethasone.
- Oral: 1 mg, 5 mg, 25 mg tablets. PLT is a compound preparation containing cinchophen.

DOSES

Dogs:

- Ophthalmic: Dosage frequency and duration of therapy is dependent upon type of lesion and response to therapy. Usually 1 drop in affected eye(s) q4–24h tapering in response to therapy.
- Hypoadrenocorticism: Starting dose 0.2 mg/kg with desoxycortone pivalate (DOCP), 0.1 mg /kg with fludrocortisone. The dose of prednisolone may be reduced considerably in most cases once the animal is stable. In cases on fludrocortisone it may be discontinued but in cases on DOCP it should be continued albeit at a low dose.
- Allergy: 0.5–1.0 mg/kg p.o. q12h initially, tapering to lowest q48h dose.
- Anti-inflammatory: 0.5 mg/kg p.o. q12–24h; taper to 0.25–0.5 mg/kg q48h.
- Immunosuppression: 1.0–2.0 mg/kg p.o. q24h, tapering slowly to 0.5 mg/kg q48h (for many conditions this will take 6 months).
- Lymphoma: see the *BSAVA Small Animal Formulary, 9th edition – Part A: Canine and Feline.*

Cats:

- Ophthalmic, Hypoadrenocorticism, Allergy: Doses as for dogs.

- Anti-inflammatory: 0.5–1.0 mg/kg p.o. q12–24h; taper to 0.5 mg/kg q48h.
- Immunosuppression: 1.0–2.0 mg/kg p.o. q12–24h, tapering slowly to 0.5–1.0 mg/kg q48h (for many conditions this will take 6 months).
- Lymphoma: see the *BSAVA Small Animal Formulary, 9th edition – Part A: Canine and Feline.*

Mammals:

- Primates: anti-inflammatory: 0.5 mg/kg p.o., s.c., i.m. q24h; allergy, autoimmune disease: up to 2 mg/kg p.o., s.c., i.m. q24h
- Sugar gliders: anti-inflammatory: 0.1–0.2 mg/kg p.o., s.c., i.m. q24h
- Hedgehogs: allergy: 2.5 mg/kg p.o., s.c., i.m. q12h
- Ferrets: lymphoma (see the *BSAVA Small Animal Formulary, 9th edition – Part B: Exotic Pets*); anti-inflammatory: 1–2 mg/kg p.o. q24h; postoperative management of adrenalectomy: 0.25–0.5 mg/kg p.o. q12h, taper to q48h
- Rabbits: anti-inflammatory: 0.25–0.5 mg/kg p.o. q12h for 3 days, then q24h for 3 days, then q48h
- Others: anti-inflammatory: 1.25–2.5 mg/kg p.o. q24h. Ophthalmic: Dosage frequency and duration of therapy is dependent upon the type of lesion and response to therapy. Usually 1 drop in the affected eye(s) q4–24h, tapering in response to therapy. Care should be exercised in rabbits, as they are highly sensitive to the effects of steroids, even in topical preparations.

Birds: Pruritus: 1 mg/kg p.o. q12h, reduced to minimum effective dose as quickly as possible.

Reptiles: Analgesic, anti-inflammatory: 2–5 mg/kg p.o. q24–48h; Lymphoma: 2 mg/kg p.o. q24h for 2 weeks, then 1 mg/kg p.o. q24h as part of the chemotherapy protocol in a Green iguana.

Amphibians, Fish: No information available.

Prescribing cascade [25, 26]

Veterinary medicinal products must be administered in accordance with the prescribing cascade, as set out in the Veterinary Medicines Regulations 2013. These Regulations provide that when no authorized veterinary medicinal product exists for a condition in a particular species, veterinary surgeons exercising their clinical judgement may, in particular to avoid unacceptable suffering, prescribe for one or a small number of animals under their care other suitable medications in accordance with the following sequence:

1. A veterinary medicine authorized in the UK for use in another animal species, or for a different condition in the same species
2. If there is no such product:
   - A medicine authorized in the UK for human use
   - A veterinary medicine not authorized in the UK, but authorized in another member state for use in any animal species in accordance with the Special Import Scheme.
3. A medicine prepared by the veterinary surgeon responsible for treating the animal and prepared especially on this occasion
4. In exceptional circumstances, medicines may be imported from outside Europe via the Special Import Scheme.

'Off-label' use of medicines

'Off-label' use is the use of medicines outside the terms of their marketing authorization. It may include medicines authorized outside the UK that are used in accordance with an import certificate issued by the VMD. A veterinary surgeon with detailed knowledge of the medical history and clinical status of a patient, may reasonably prescribe a medicine 'off-label' in accordance with the prescribing cascade. Authorized medicines have been scientifically assessed against statutory criteria of safety, quality and efficacy when used in accordance with the authorized recommendations on the product literature. Use of an unauthorized medicine provides none of these safeguards and may, therefore, pose potential risks that the authorization process seeks to minimize.

Medicines may be used 'off-label' for a variety of reasons including:

- No authorized product is suitable for the condition or specific subpopulation being treated
- Need to alter the duration of therapy, dosage, route of administration, etc., to treat the specific condition presented
- An authorized product has proved ineffective in the circumstances of a particular case (all cases of suspected lack of efficacy of authorized veterinary medicines should be reported to the VMD).

Responsibility for the use of a medicine 'off-label' lies solely with the prescribing veterinary surgeon.

He or she should inform the owner of the reason why a medicine is to be used 'off-label' and record this reason in the patient's clinical notes. When electing to use a medicine 'off-label' always:

- Discuss all therapeutic options with the owner
- Use the cascade to determine your choice of medicine
- Obtain signed informed consent if an unauthorized product is to be used, ensuring that all potential problems are explained to the client
- Administer unauthorized medicines against a patient-specific prescription. Do not administer to a group of animals if at all possible.

An 'off-label' medicine must show a comparative clinical advantage to the authorized product in the specific circumstances presented (where applicable).

Medicines may be used 'off-label' in the following ways (this is not an exhaustive list):

- Authorized product at an unauthorized dose
- Authorized product for an unauthorized indication
- Authorized product used outwith the authorized age range
- Authorized product administered by an unauthorized route
- Authorized product used to treat an animal in an unauthorized physiological state, e.g. pregnancy (i.e. an unauthorized indication)
- Product authorized for use in humans or a different animal species to that being treated.

Adverse effects may or may not be specific for a species, and idiosyncratic reactions are always a possibility. If no adverse effects are listed, consider data from different species. When using novel or unfamiliar drugs, consider pharmaceutical and pharmacological interactions. In some species, and with some diseases, the ability to metabolize/ excrete a drug may be impaired/enhanced. Use the lowest dose that might be effective and the safest route of administration. Ensure that you are aware of the clinical signs that may suggest toxicity.

NOTES

Prescription – standard form [25]

From: Address of practice   Date
Telephone No.
Animal's name and identification   Owner's name
(species, breed, age and sex)   Owner's address

Rx   Print name, strength and formulation of drug

     Total quantity to be supplied

     Amount to be administered

     Frequency of administration

     Duration of treatment

     Any warnings

     If not a POM-V and prescribed under the 'Cascade', this must
     be stated

     For animal treatment only

     For an animal under my care

Non-repeat/repeat x 1, 2 or 3

       Name, qualifications and signature of veterinary surgeon

NOTES

Pruritus – cat [11]

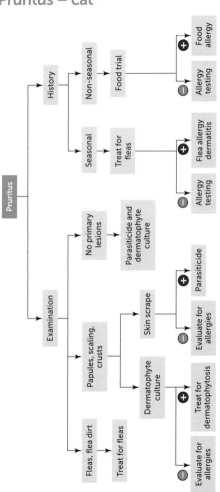

Diagnostic approach to a pruritic cat.

Pruritus – dog [11]

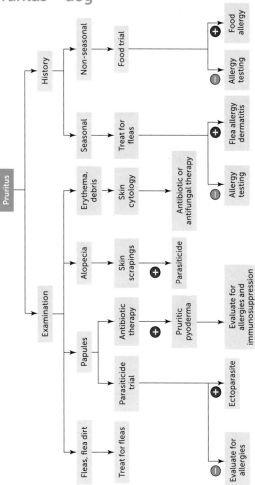

Diagnostic approach to a pruritic dog.

Pruritus scale [11]

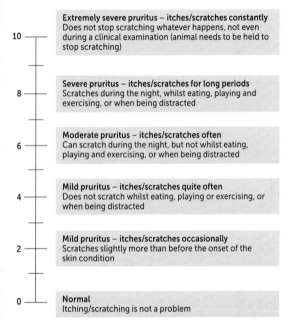

10	**Extremely severe pruritus – itches/scratches constantly** Does not stop scratching whatever happens, not even during a clinical examination (animal needs to be held to stop scratching)
8	**Severe pruritus – itches/scratches for long periods** Scratches during the night, whilst eating, playing and exercising, or when being distracted
6	**Moderate pruritus – itches/scratches often** Can scratch during the night, but not whilst eating, playing and exercising, or when being distracted
4	**Mild pruritus – itches/scratches quite often** Does not scratch whilst eating, playing or exercising, or when being distracted
2	**Mild pruritus – itches/scratches occasionally** Scratches slightly more than before the onset of the skin condition
0	**Normal** Itching/scratching is not a problem

The owner marks the bar at the appropriate level. This will give an estimated pruritus score (0–10) for the animal.

NOTES

NOTES

Pyoderma – investigation of clinical signs [11]

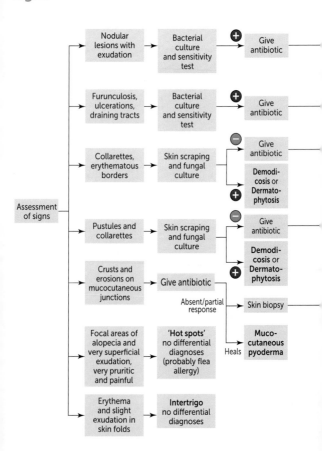

GSD = German Shepherd Dog.

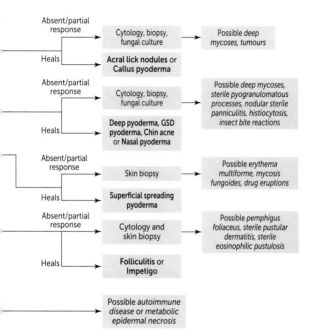

Absent/partial response → Cytology, biopsy, fungal culture → Possible *deep mycoses, tumours*

Heals → **Acral lick nodules** or **Callus pyoderma**

Absent/partial response → Cytology, biopsy, fungal culture → Possible *deep mycoses, sterile pyogranulomatous processes, nodular sterile panniculitis, histiocytosis, insect bite reactions*

Heals → **Deep pyoderma, GSD pyoderma, Chin acne** or **Nasal pyoderma**

Absent/partial response → Skin biopsy → Possible *erythema multiforme, mycosis fungoides, drug eruptions*

Heals → **Superficial spreading pyoderma**

Absent/partial response → Cytology and skin biopsy → Possible *pemphigus foliaceus, sterile pustular dermatitis, sterile eosinophilic pustulosis*

Heals → **Folliculitis** or **Impetigo**

→ Possible *autoimmune disease* or *metabolic epidermal necrosis*

Pyrantel [25, 26]
(Cazitel, Cestem, Dolpac, Droncit, Drontal, Endoguard, Prazitel, Veloxa, Various other preparations) POM-V

Formulations: Oral: Pyrantel with praziquantel and febantel (50 mg, 50 mg, 150 mg; 175 mg, 175 mg, 525 mg) tablets; pyrantel with praziquantel and oxantel (10 mg, 10 mg, 40 mg; 25 mg, 25 mg, 100 mg; 50 mg, 50 mg, 200 mg; 125 mg, 125 mg, 500 mg) tablets; 5 mg/ml liquid; pyrantel embonate with praziquantel (230 mg, 20 mg; 345 mg, 30 mg) tablets; 14.4 mg/ml pyrantel embonate with 15 mg/ml febantel suspension.

Note: some formulations and doses give content of pyrantel (febantel, oxantel) in terms of pyrantel embonate/pamonate (50 mg pyrantel is equivalent to 144 mg pyrantel embonate/pamonate).

DOSES

Dogs: 5 mg/kg pyrantel + 15 mg/kg febantel or 20 mg/kg oxantel p.o., repeat as required.

Cats: 57.5 mg/kg pyrantel embonate.

Mammals:
- Primates: 11 mg/kg p.o., repeat in 14 days
- Ferrets: 4.4 mg/kg (pyrantel embonate) p.o., repeat in 14 days
- Rabbits: 5–10 mg/kg (pyrantel embonate/pamoate) p.o., repeat in 10–21 days
- Rodents: 50 mg/kg (pyrantel embonate/pamoate) p.o., repeat as required.

Reptiles: 5 mg/kg p.o., repeat in 14 days has been suggested for the treatment of endoparasites.

Amphibians: 5 mg/kg p.o. q14d.

Birds, Fish: No Information available.

NOTES

NOTES

Rabbit biological data [21]

Lifespan (years)	5–12 (can be greater in some individuals)
Average weight (kg)	1–10 (breed-dependent)
Heart rate (beats/min)	180–300
Respiratory rate (breaths/min)	30–60 (higher if stressed)
Blood volume (ml/kg)	Approximately 60
Rectal temperature (°C)	38.5–40.0
Dentition	I2/1 C0/0 P3/2 M3/3
Daily water intake (ml/kg)	50–150
Daily urine production (ml/kg)	10–35
Food intake per day (g/kg)	50
Sexual maturity	4–8 months (does earlier than bucks)
Oestrous cycle	Induced (reflex) ovulation; oestrus January–October
Length of gestation (days)	28–32
Litter size	4–12
Birth weight (g)	30–80
Weaning age (weeks)	6

NOTES

Rabbit reproduction – common owner concerns [23]

- **Accidental mating:** If a litter is not wanted, consider spaying in early stages of pregnancy or giving aglepristone.
- **Pregnancy diagnosis:** Via ultrasonography at 6+ days, radiographically at 11+ days or by palpation at 10–12 days by an experienced person.
- **Length of gestation:** Average 31 days, range 30–33 days.
- **Delivery:** Does will often give birth at night or early in the morning, so all that is seen by the owner are a few spots of blood and a moving nest of fur.
- **Re-mating:** The doe is fertile immediately after giving birth so entire male companions should be removed. If they are not the doe will very likely go on to produce a second litter a month later. In rare cases delayed implantation may occur.
- **Difficult deliveries:** It is very unusual to witness a doe in labour. Early signs include pulling fur. A doe observed straining or with visible spots of blood in the absence of kits is likely to be experiencing difficulty. The need for veterinary intervention is indicated.
- **Feeding:** Does feed their kits once or at most twice daily; this is rarely witnessed. For this reason owners often assume that a litter is being neglected.
  - It is not always possible to tell whether kits are being fed in the first 48 hours, therefore they should only be removed from the doe if she is harming them or too unwell to care for them.
  - If after 48 hours the kits are unfed the skin will be wrinkled owing to dehydration, they may feel cool to touch and be weak. Now is the time to decide whether to start supplementary feeding or hand-rearing.
  - Kits 2–5 days old may still be very active and vocal when touched; it is not unusual for them to be hungry at this stage, especially if it is a large litter.

- **Kits:** Altricial, i.e. born blind, naked and helpless.
  - Kits should not be handled in the first few days other than to check they are alive.
  - Eyes open at 10–12 days.
  - Kits start to leave the nest any time after the eyes open. The longer the kits stay in the nest the better fed they are. Some kits will not be seen until nearly 3 weeks of age.
  - Daily handling of kits from the time they leave the nest is good but only for very short periods to begin with.
- **Sexing:** Best done at 4 weeks of age; between 6 and 10 weeks it can be a little more awkward. If an experienced examiner is finding it difficult to determine the sex, the possibility of a buck with hypospadias should be considered. These males will often appear to be female and it can be difficult to be sure of their sex until the testes descend.

Rabbits – anorexia *see* Anorexia in rabbits

NOTES

Ranitidine [25,26]

(Ranitidine*, Zantac*) POM

Formulations:

- Injectable: 25 mg/ml solution
- Oral: 75 mg, 150 mg, 300 mg tablets; 15 mg/ml syrup.

DOSES

Dogs: 2 mg/kg slow i.v., s.c., p.o. q8–12h.

Cats: 2 mg/kg/day constant i.v. infusion, 2.5 mg/kg i.v. slowly q12h, 3.5 mg/kg p.o. q12h.

Mammals:

- Primates: 0.5 mg/kg p.o. q24h (anti-ulcer)
- Ferrets: 3.5 mg/kg p.o. q12h; Rabbits: 4–6 mg/kg p.o., s.c. q8–24h
- Chinchillas, Guinea pigs: 5 mg/kg p.o. q12h as a prokinetic.

Birds, Reptiles, Amphibians, Fish: No information available.

Rat biological data [21]

Lifespan (years)	2–3.5
Adult bodyweight (g)	Males: 270–500 Females: 225–325
Dentition	2 [I1/1 C0/0 P0/0 M3/3] Only incisors open-rooted
Number of digits	Front: 4 Rear: 5
Rectal temperature (°C)	~38
Heart rate (beats/min)	310–500
Respiratory rate (breaths/min)	70–150
Environmental temperature (°C)	21–24
Relative humidity (%)	45–55
Daily water intake	10 ml/100 g

Fluid therapy	101 ml/kg/24h
Diet	Omnivorous
Food intake per day per animal (g)	15–20
Coprophagy/Caecotrophy?	Yes
Oestrous type	Continuous polyoestrous
Post-partum oestrus?	Yes
Age at puberty (months)	1
Gestation length (days)	21–23
Oestrous cycle (days)	4–5
Oestrus duration (hours)	9–20
Litter size	6–13
Birth weight (g)	4–6
Altricial/Precocial	Altricial
Eyes open (days)	12–15
Age at weaning (days)	21
Number of pairs of teats	6
Minimum breeding age (months)	2
Ratio for breeding (M:F)	1:1–6 If polygamous remove female on day 16
Comments	They will eat the litter if disturbed in the first 2–3 days

NOTES

Respiratory distress [8]

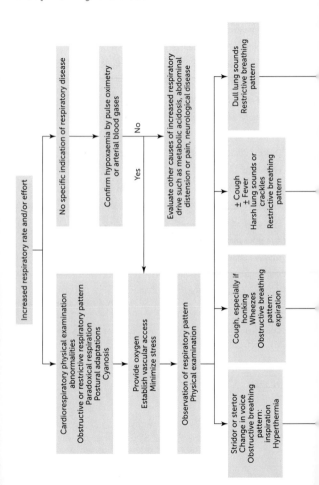

Increased respiratory rate and/or effort

No specific indication of respiratory disease

Confirm hypoxaemia by pulse oximetry or arterial blood gases

Yes — No

Evaluate other causes of increased respiratory drive such as metabolic acidosis, abdominal distension or pain, neurological disease

Cardiorespiratory physical examination abnormalities
Obstructive or restrictive respiratory pattern
Paradoxical respiration
Postural adaptations
Cyanosis

Provide oxygen
Establish vascular access
Minimize stress

Observation of respiratory pattern
Physical examination

Dull lung sounds
Restrictive breathing pattern

± Cough
± Fever
Harsh lung sounds or crackles
Restrictive breathing pattern

Cough, especially if honking
Wheezes
Obstructive breathing pattern: expiration

Stridor or stertor
Change in voice
Obstructive breathing pattern: inspiration
Hyperthermia

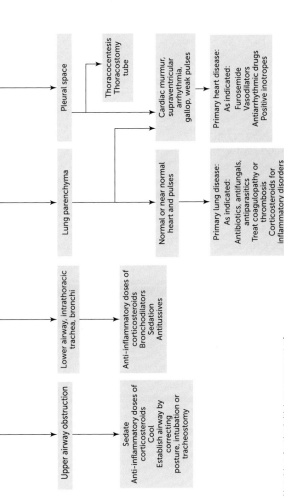

Algorithm for the initial management of animals with respiratory distress.

Upper airway obstruction → Sedate
Anti-inflammatory doses of corticosteroids
Cool
Establish airway by correcting posture, intubation or tracheostomy

Lower airway, intrathoracic trachea, bronchi → Anti-inflammatory doses of corticosteroids
Bronchodilators
Sedation
Antitussives

Lung parenchyma → Normal or near normal heart and pulses → Primary lung disease:
As indicated:
Antibiotics, antifungals, antiparasitics
Treat coagulopathy or thrombosis
Corticosteroids for inflammatory disorders

Pleural space → Thoracocentesis
Thoracostomy tube

Cardiac murmur, supraventricular arrhythmia, gallop, weak pulses → Primary heart disease:
As indicated:
Furosemide
Vasodilators
Antiarrhythmic drugs
Positive inotropes

Resting energy requirement (RER) [12]

Interspecific formulae	Feline formula
RER = 70 $(Wt_{kg})^{0.75}$ RER = 30 (Wt_{kg}) + 70	RER = 40 (Wt_{kg})

The interspecific formulae tend to overestimate feline energy requirements. Wt = bodyweight.

Robenacoxib [25]
(Onsior) POM-V

Formulations:
- Oral: 5 mg, 10 mg, 20 mg, 40 mg flavoured tablets for dogs; 6 mg flavoured tablets for cats.
- Injectable: 20 mg/ml solution.

DOSES

Dogs, Cats: 2 mg/kg s.c. q24h for a maximum of 2 doses; 1–2 mg/kg p.o. q24h (in cats for up to 6 days).

Onsior (from datasheet)					
Dose rate	Bodyweight (kg)	No. of tablets per day			
		5 mg	10 mg	20 mg	40 mg
Dogs					
1–2 mg/kg q24h	2.5–<5	1			
	5–<10		1		
	10–<20			1	
	20–<40				1
	40–80				2

NOTES

NOTES

Schirmer tear test [16]

Dogs:

- Normal = >15 mm/minute
- Early/subclinical keratoconjunctivitis sicca (KCS) = 10–15 mm/minute. These readings are equivocal and testing should be repeated at a later date
- Mild/moderate KCS = 6–9 mm/minute. Values <10 mm/minute are diagnostic for KCS in conjunction with compatible clinical signs
- Severe KCS = ≤5 mm/minute

Cats: Normal = 3–32 mm/minute (mean of 17 mm/minute).

NOTES

Sedation combinations [7, 26]

For dogs and cats

Drug combination	
Drug 1	*Drug 2*
Acepromazine (0.03–0.05 mg/kg)	+ Buprenorphine (20 µg/kg) + Butorphanol (0.2–0.4 mg/kg) + Hydromorphone (0.1–0.2 mg/kg) + Methadone (0.2–0.5 mg/kg) + Morphine (0.2–0.5 mg/kg) + Pethidine (meperidine) (4–5 mg/kg)
Dexmedetomidine (1–10 µg/kg) Use 1–3 µg/kg i.v. Doses up to 10 µg/kg may be used i.m. if profound sedation is required	+ Buprenorphine (20 µg/kg) + Butorphanol (0.2–0.4 mg/kg) + Hydromorphone (0.1–0.15 mg/kg) + Methadone (0.1–0.2 mg/kg) + Morphine (0.1–0.2 mg/kg) + Pethidine (4–5 mg/kg)
Dexmedetomidine (1–10 µg/kg) Use 1–3 µg/kg i.v. Doses up to 10 µg/kg may be used i.m. if profound sedation is required	+ Diazepam (0.3 mg/kg) + Midazolam (0.3 mg/kg)
Midazolam (0.4–0.5 mg/kg)	+ Hydromorphone (0.1–0.15 mg/kg) + Methadone (0.2–0.5 mg/kg) + Morphine (0.2–0.5 mg/kg)

Route of administration	Species notes	Sedation notes
i.m. or i.v. i.m. or i.v. i.m. or i.v. i.m. or i.v. i.m. i.m.	Cat: use low to mid-dose range of opioids Dog: higher doses of opioids will provide greater sedation	Will provide light sedation in cats and dogs. Do not expect animals to become recumbent. Use lower end of dose range when drugs are given i.v.
i.m. or i.v. i.m. or i.v. i.m. or i.v. i.m. or i.v. i.m. i.m.	Cat and dog	Higher doses of dexmedetomidine will provide more reliable and profound sedation. Expect animals to become recumbent. Useful for minor invasive painful procedures such as removal of grass seeds from the ear canal. Use lower end of dose range when drugs are given i.v.
i.v. i.m. or i.v.	Cat and dog	Higher doses of dexmedetomidine will provide more reliable and profound sedation. Expect animals to become recumbent. Degree of analgesia is less than when dexmedetomidine is combined with an opioid. Use lower end of dose range when drugs are given i.v.
i.m. or i.v. i.m. or i.v. i.m.	Dog	Degree of sedation will depend on the health and temperament of the patient. May be able to carry out some invasive procedures if the animal is handled patiently and quietly. Use lower end of dose range when drugs are given i.v. ⟶

Drug combination		
Drug 1	*Drug 2*	
Midazolam (0.2–0.3 mg/kg)	+ Ketamine (2–5 mg/kg)	
Zolazepam + tiletamine	Available as a proprietary mixture (Telazol® or Zoletil®). Dose range for sedation/ short-duration general anaesthesia: 9–13 mg/kg	
Alfaxalone (1–3 mg/kg) Use lower end of dose range when administering i.m. or in combination with other drugs. Use higher dose s.c.	+ Buprenorphine (20 µg/kg) + Butorphanol (0.2–0.4 mg/kg) + Methadone (0.2–0.5 mg/kg)	
Alfaxalone (0.2–0.5 mg/kg i.v.)	+ Butorphanol (0.2–0.3 mg/kg) or midazolam (0.2–0.3 mg/kg)	
Morphine (0.2–0.5 mg/kg) Methadone (0.2–0.5 mg/kg) Hydromorphone (0.1–0.15 mg/kg)		

For exotic pets

Ferrets:

- Ketamine (5–8 µg (micrograms)/kg i.m.) plus medetomidine (80–100 µg/kg i.m.) or dexmedetomidine (40–50 µg/kg i.m.) to which can be added butorphanol (0.1–0.2 mg/kg i.m.) or buprenorphine (0.02 mg/kg i.m.).

Route of administration	Species notes	Sedation notes
i.m. or i.v.	Cat	Expect profound sedation/light general anaesthesia. Use lower end of dose range when drugs are given i.v.
i.m. or i.v.	Cat and dog	As above for midazolam/ketamine mixture. Recovery can be stormy in dogs. Use lower end of dose range when drugs are given i.v.
i.m. or s.c. i.m. or s.c. i.m. or s.c.	Cat and dog	Volume limits utility in most dogs. Midazolam (0.2–0.3 mg/kg) may be added to this combination to provide increased sedation in anxious or fearful cats and dogs
i.v.	Cat and dog	For (non-painful) diagnostic procedures, start with lower dose, dilute with sterile water for injection or saline to ensure more accurate dosing and have means to intubate within reach
i.m. i.m. or i.v. i.m. or i.v.	Cat and dog	Mild sedation only. Do not expect animal to become recumbent. Use lower end of dose range when drugs are given i.v.

- Ketamine (5–20 mg/kg i.m.) plus midazolam (0.25–0.5 mg/kg i.m.) or diazepam (0.25–0.5 mg/kg i.m.) will provide immobilization or, at the higher doses, a short period of anaesthesia.
- Ketamine (7–10 mg/kg i.m., s.c.) plus medetomidine (20 µg (micrograms)/kg i.m., s.c.) plus midazolam (0.5 mg/kg i.m., s.c.) will provide anaesthesia; concurrent oxygenation is recommended.

⟩⟩⟩

Rabbits:

■ Ketamine (3–5 mg/kg i.v. or 5–10 mg/kg i.m., s.c.) in combination with medetomidine (0.05–0.1 mg/kg i.v. or 0.1–0.3 mg/kg s.c., i.m.) or dexmedetomidine (0.025–0.05 mg/kg i.v. or 0.05–0.15 mg/kg s.c., i.m.) and butorphanol (0.05–0.1 mg/kg i.m., i.v., s.c.) or buprenorphine (0.02–0.05 mg/kg i.m., i.v., s.c.).

■ Fentanyl/fluanisone (0.1–0.3 ml/kg i.m.) plus diazepam (0.5–1 mg/kg i.v., i.m. or 2.5–5.0 mg/kg intraperitoneal) or midazolam (0.25–1.0 mg/kg i.v., i.m., intraperitoneal).

■ The combinations above will provide immobilization/light anaesthesia, usually sufficient to allow intubation for maintenance with a volatile agent.

■ Ketamine (15 mg/kg i.m.) in combination with medetomidine (0.25 mg/kg i.m.) and buprenorphine (0.03 mg/kg i.m.) will provide general anaesthesia, but use of lower doses followed by intubation and use of a volatile agent is recommended.

Other small mammals:

■ Medetomidine (50 µg (micrograms)/kg i.m.) or dexmedetomidine (25 µg/kg i.m.) plus, if needed, ketamine (2–4 mg/kg i.m.).

■ Other combinations as for rabbits. Combinations can also be administered intraperitoneal in small rodents.

Note: Reduce doses if animal is debilitated. For all small mammals, for deeper anaesthesia, intubation (if possible) and use of a volatile agent is recommended, rather than using higher doses of injectable agents.

For information on Sedation protocols in birds, reptiles and fish, see the *BSAVA Small Animal Formulary – Part B: Exotic Pets*.

See also Acepromazine, Buprenorphine, Butorphanol, Dexmedetomidine, Diazepam, Ketamine, Medetomidine ***and*** Methadone

NOTES

Sedation of fractious dogs and cats [7]

Drug combination	
Drug 1	Drug 1
Dexmedeto-midine (10 µg/kg)	+ Butorphanol (0.4–0.5 mg/kg) + Methadone (0.4–0.5 mg/kg) + Hydromorphone (0.1–0.15 mg/kg)
Dexmedeto-midine (20–40 µg/kg)	+ Buprenorphine (20 µg/kg) Use preservative-free preparation of buprenorphine
Ketamine (5 mg/kg)	+ Midazolam (0.3 mg/kg) and butorphanol (0.3 mg/kg) + Midazolam (0.3 mg/kg) and methadone (0.3 mg/kg) + Midazolam (0.3 mg/kg) and hydromorphone (0.1 mg/kg)
Alfaxalone (2–3 mg/kg)	+ Midazolam (0.2–0.3 mg/kg) and methadone (0.3–0.4 mg/kg) + Midazolam (0.2–0.3 mg/kg) and hydromorphone (0.1 mg/kg) + Midazolam (0.2–0.3 mg/kg) and butorphanol (0.3–0.4 mg/kg)
Acepromazine (0.1 mg/kg)	+ Midazolam (0.3 mg/kg) and methadone (0.5 mg/kg) + Midazolam (0.3 mg/kg) and hydromorphone (0.1 mg/kg)
Sevoflurane	

Drug combinations used for sedation and pre-anaesthetic medication of fractious or fearful cats and dogs when intravenous access is not established.

Route of administration	Species	Patient selection
i.m.	Cat and dog	This dose of dexmedetomidine will cause significant cardiovascular depression; best reserved for use in healthy animals. Use methadone in animals undergoing painful interventions
OTM	Cat	Use the higher dose of dexmedetomidine in feral cats; the lower dose will usually be sufficient in cats that are only very nervous
i.m.	Cat	Use methadone in animals undergoing painful interventions. May be a useful alternative to combinations with dexmedetomidine in animals that cannot be examined before drug administration and are of unknown health status. Avoid ketamine in cats with hypertrophic cardiomyopathy
i.m. or s.c. Use lower dose when administering i.m., use higher dose s.c.	Cat and dog	Volume required limits utility in most dogs. May be a useful combination in cats with hypertrophic cardiomyopathy that are unsuitable for either dexmedetomidine or ketamine administration
i.m. or s.c.	Dog	Produces less reliable sedation than combinations incorporating dexmedetomidine
Administer via an induction chamber	Cat	Induction of anaesthesia using sevoflurane can be unpleasant for cats but this technique can be useful if i.m. drug administration proves impossible. Alternatively, it can be used to provide 'top-up' sedation to allow i.v. access in cats that are not adequately sedated after i.m. administration of sedative drugs

Seizures **see** Status epilepticus

Selamectin [25, 26]
(Stronghold) POM-V

Formulations: Topical: Spot-on pipettes, 5 sizes for dogs, 2 sizes for cats, containing 6% or 12% selamectin.

DOSES

Dogs, Cats: Parasiticide: Minimum dose recommendation 6 mg/kg. For flea and heartworm prevention apply monthly. For the treatment of roundworms, lice and ear mites one application. For effective treatment of sarcoptic mange apply product on three occasions at 2-week intervals.

Mammals: Sugar gliders, Hedgehogs: 6 mg/kg monthly; Ferrets, Rabbits, Rodents: 6–15 mg/kg monthly.

Birds, Reptiles, Amphibians, Fish: No information available.

Shock — classification scheme [12]

Broad category	Type of shock	Definition
Circulatory	Hypovolaemic	Decreased intravascular volume
	Cardiogenic	Reduced cardiac output ('forward' or 'pump' failure)
	Obstructive	Physical obstruction to blood flow leading, ultimately, to reduced filling of the left side of the heart (heart and/or great vessels)
	Distributive	Maldistribution of blood flow (vasodilatation, vasoconstriction)
Non-circulatory	Hypoxic	Decreased oxygen content in arterial blood (anaemia, hypoxaemia, dyshaemoglobinaemia)
	Metabolic	Impaired cellular metabolism

Shock — general approach to diagnostic testing [12]

All patients

- Major body system assessment and full physical examination
- Placement of ECG leads for monitoring heart rate and rhythm
- Non-invasive arterial blood pressure measurement
- S_pO_2 measurement
- Blood sampling from the intravenous catheter at placement:
  - Blood from the hub of the catheter can be used to run an emergency database (PCV, TS, blood glucose, BUN, blood smear)
- Where it is possible to collect further blood samples at placement without compromising the catheter, consider:
  - Cage-side venous blood gas, electrolyte, lactate measurement (typically only 0.1–0.2 ml of blood required)
  - Filling a serum gel and EDTA blood tube and reserving for later haematology and biochemistry panels

Selected patients

- 3-lead ECG measurement in patients with tachycardia, bradycardia or a suspected arrhythmia
- Ultrasound examination of the abdomen and/or pleural and pericardial spaces for free fluid (Point-of-care ultrasound scan (POCUS)) in patients in which fluid accumulation is suspected based on clinical history, examination or results of the emergency database (e.g. low PCV/TS with no evidence of external haemorrhage)
- Diagnostic abdominocentesis, thoracocentesis or pericardiocentesis if required (thoracocentesis and pericardiocentesis may also be therapeutic)
- Radiography is almost always delayed until after initial stabilization, with rare exceptions (e.g. GDV) where a rapid radiographic diagnosis is required
- Blood collection for blood typing if anaemia is suspected, or coagulation panel if a coagulopathy is suspected

BUN = blood urea nitrogen; ECG = electrocardiogram; EDTA = ethylenediaminetetraacetic acid; GDV = gastric dilatation–volvulus; PCV = packed cell volume; S_pO_2 = peripheral capillary oxygen saturation; TS = total solids.

Skin lesions [5]

Primary lesions

- Macule – non-palpable area of different colour, <1 cm diameter
- Patch – macule >1 cm diameter
- Papule – solid elevation <1 cm diameter
- Nodule – solid elevation >1 cm diameter
- Plaque – platform-like elevation
- Vesicle – blister <1 cm, filled with clear fluid
- Bulla – blister >1 cm
- Pustule – vesicle filled with pus
- Tumour – large mass
- Wheal – raised, oedematous area (pitting on pressure)

Primary or secondary lesions

- Alopecia – loss of hair: spontaneous alopecia is primary; self-induced alopecia is secondary
- Scale – flakes of cornified cells
- Crust – dried exudate containing blood/serum/scales/pus
- Follicular casts – accumulation of keratin and follicular material like a sock around the base of the hair shaft
- Comedo – hair follicle plugged with keratin and sebum
- Hyperpigmentation – increased pigmentation
- Hypopigmentation – decreased pigmentation

Secondary lesions

- Collarette – circular, peeling lesion (often a remnant of a pustule)
- Scar – fibrous tissue replacing damaged dermis/subcutis
- Erosion – epidermal defect, not extending beneath the basement membrane
- Ulcer – skin defect below the level of the basement membrane
- Fissure – deep split
- Lichenification – thickening and hardening of the skin
- Excoriation – mild erosions caused by self-trauma

NOTES

Spinal trauma [15]

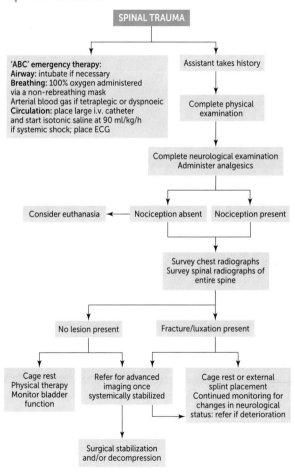

An approach to the management of spinal trauma.

Spinosad [25]
(Comfortis, Trifexis) POM-V

Formulations: Oral: 90 mg, 140 mg, 270 mg, 425 mg, 665 mg, 1040 mg, 1620 mg chewable tablets. Also available with milbemycin (Trifexis).

DOSES

Dogs: Fleas 45–70 mg/kg p.o. q28d with or immediately after food.

Cats: Fleas 50–75 mg/kg p.o. q28d with or immediately after food.

Comfortis (from datasheet)									
Dose rate	Patient bodyweight (kg)	No. of tablets required							
		90 mg	140 mg	180 mg	270 mg	425 mg	665 mg	1040 mg	1620 mg
Dogs									
45–70 mg/ kg q28d	1.3–2	1							
	2.1–3		1						
	3.1–3.8			1					
	3.9–6				1				
	6.1–9.4					1			
	9.5–14.7						1		
	14.8–23.1							1	
	23.2–36								1
	36.1–50.7						1		1
	50.8–72								2
Cats									
50–75 mg/ kg q28d	1.2–1.8	1							
	1.9–2.8		1						
	2.9–3.6			1					
	3.7–5.4				1				
	5.5–8.5 [a]					1			

[a]Cats over 8.5 kg: give the appropriate combination of tablets.

Status epilepticus [15]

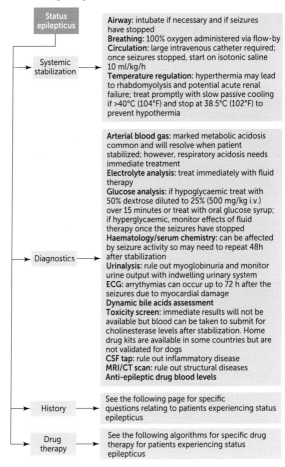

Status epilepticus

Systemic stabilization

Airway: intubate if necessary and if seizures have stopped
Breathing: 100% oxygen administered via flow-by
Circulation: large intravenous catheter required; once seizures stopped, start on isotonic saline 10 ml/kg/h
Temperature regulation: hyperthermia may lead to rhabdomyolysis and potential acute renal failure; treat promptly with slow passive cooling if >40°C (104°F) and stop at 38.5°C (102°F) to prevent hypothermia

Diagnostics

Arterial blood gas: marked metabolic acidosis common and will resolve when patient stabilized; however, respiratory acidosis needs immediate treatment
Electrolyte analysis: treat immediately with fluid therapy
Glucose analysis: if hypoglycaemic treat with 50% dextrose diluted to 25% (500 mg/kg i.v.) over 15 minutes or treat with oral glucose syrup; if hyperglycaemic, monitor effects of fluid therapy once the seizures have stopped
Haematology/serum chemistry: can be affected by seizure activity so may need to repeat 48h after stabilization
Urinalysis: rule out myoglobinuria and monitor urine output with indwelling urinary system
ECG: arrythmias can occur up to 72 h after the seizures due to myocardial damage
Dynamic bile acids assessment
Toxicity screen: immediate results will not be available but blood can be taken to submit for cholinesterase levels after stabilization. Home drug kits are available in some countries but are not validated for dogs
CSF tap: rule out inflammatory disease
MRI/CT scan: rule out structural diseases
Anti-epileptic drug blood levels

History

See the following page for specific questions relating to patients experiencing status epilepticus

Drug therapy

See the following algorithms for specific drug therapy for patients experiencing status epilepticus

Approach to systemic stabilization and management of the status epilepticus patient.

- When did the episode start?
- Is there a pre-existing seizure disorder?
- Has the patient had status epilepticus or cluster seizure events before?
- Have there been any systemic health problems within the last 4 months?
- Has there been any change in the patient's personality or behaviour within the last 4 months?
- Is the patient on any medication, including anticonvulsant therapy?
- Which anticonvulsants are being given; what is the dose; when was the last dose?
- How long has the patient been on anticonvulsants?
- Have recent serum anticonvulsant measurements been performed?
- Is there any recent trauma, travel history or toxin exposure?
- Has the patient eaten a meal within the last few hours?

Important questions to ask about the patient in status epilepticus.

NOTES

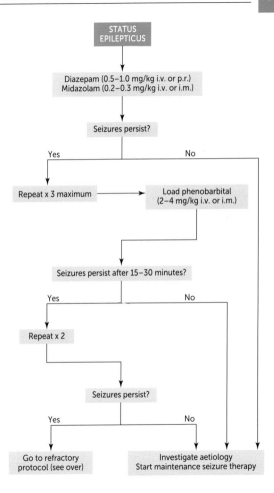

Approach to the initial pharmacological management of the status epilepticus patient.

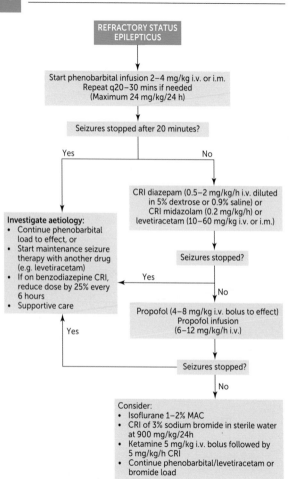

Approach to the pharmacological management of the refractory status epilepticus patient.

Sucralfate [25,26]
(Antepsin*, Antepsin suspension*, Carafate*) POM

Formulations: Oral: 1 g tablet; 0.2 g/ml suspension.

DOSES

Dogs: 500 mg/dog p.o. q6–8h (dogs up to 20 kg);
1–2 g/dog p.o. q6–8h (>20 kg).

Cats: 250 mg/cat p.o. q8–12h.

Mammals:
- Primates: 0.5 g/animal p.o. q 6–12h
- Hedgehogs: 10 mg/kg p.o. q8–12h
- Ferrets: 25–125 mg/kg p.o. q6–12h
- Rabbits: 25 mg/kg p.o. q8–12h
- Rodents: 25–50 mg/kg p.o. q6–8h.

Birds: 25 mg/kg p.o. q8h.

Reptiles: 500–1000 mg/kg p.o. q6–8h.

Amphibians, Fish: No information available.

NOTES

Suture patterns [18]

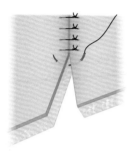

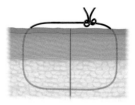

The appearance of the knot relative to the incision.

Simple interrupted suture pattern.

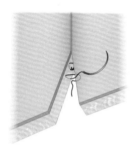

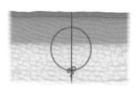

Buried intradermal knot.

Interrupted intradermal suture pattern.

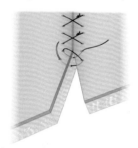

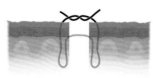

Gambee suture.

Interrupted cruciate suture pattern.

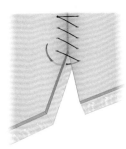

Standard simple continuous suture pattern.

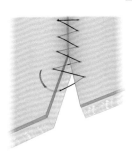

Running simple continuous suture pattern.

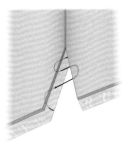

Continuous intradermal (mattress) suture pattern.

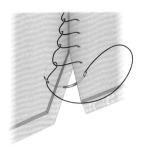

Ford interlocking suture pattern.

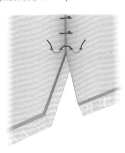

Lembert suture pattern.

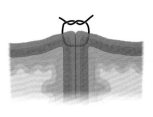

Note how this suture inverts the tissues.

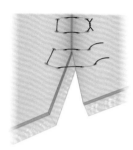

Halstead suture pattern.

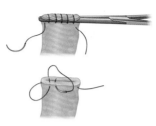

Parker-Kerr oversew. The top picture shows suturing over the haemostat with a Cushing pattern while the bottom shows the Lembert oversew.

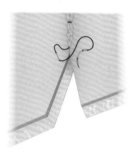

Utrecht suture pattern.

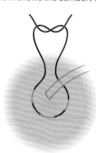

Purse-string suture.

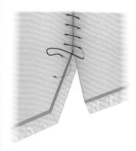

Cushing suture pattern.

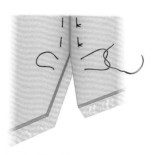

Horizontal mattress suture pattern.

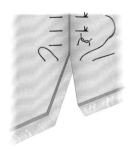

Vertical mattress suture pattern.

Suture sizes [6]

Metric (Ph. Eur.)	USP
0.5	7/0
0.7	6/0
1	5/0
1.5	4/0
2	3/0
3	2/0
3.5	0
4	1
5	2
6	3

NOTES

NOTES

Telmisartan [25]
(Semintra) POM-V

Formulations: Oral: 4 mg/ml solution.

DOSES

Dogs: No information available.

Cats: 1 mg/kg p.o. q24h.

Thiamazole *see* Methimazole

NOTES

Thoracocentesis [12]

Indications

- Patients with respiratory distress and dull lung sounds on auscultation
- Patients that present with dyspnoea after trauma (road traffic accident, bite wounds, falling from height)
- Patients that are undergoing positive pressure ventilation with sudden deterioration

Contraindications

- Severe coagulopathy

Procedure

Position the patient, preferably in sternal recumbency or standing. Lateral recumbency is also acceptable for pneumothorax. An assistant should be available to restrain the patient or give sedation as needed. In many cats a minimal restraint technique is preferred and is generally better tolerated.

1. Clip and aseptically prepare appropriate rib space:
   - If expecting fluid, the 7th or 8th intercostal space, at approximately the level of the costochondral junction
   - If expecting air, the 8th or 9th intercostal space, approximately one-third of the way down the chest.
2. Use sterile gloves for the insertion of the appropriate size needle or butterfly catheter:
   - Large dogs – 40 mm needle or even longer catheter
   - Medium sized dogs and large cats – 25 mm needle or catheter
   - Cats and small dogs – 18–22 mm butterfly needle.
3. Insert the needle slowly just cranial to the rib to avoid the intercostal blood vessels.
4. Observe the hub of the needle for any signs of fluid:
   - If a small amount of frank blood is aspirated or if the lungs can be felt rubbing against the needle, the needle should be withdrawn and moved to a different location
   - If a large amount of blood is obtained, place 1–2 ml in an empty blood collection tube to see if it clots. Blood from haemothorax should not clot, while blood from the heart or a blood vessel should clot normally, if the patient does not have a significant coagulopathy
   - For any other fluid, aspiration should continue until no more can be removed.
5. Directing the needle ventrally, rolling the patient slightly to the side on which thoracocentesis is being performed, and re-aspirating from a more ventral location can facilitate removal of as much fluid as possible.

Procedure *continued*

6. Fluid is retained for fluid analysis, cytology and possibly culture.
7. Aspiration of air will turn the tubing a slightly foggy, white colour as the warm air from the thoracic cavity encounters the room-temperature tubing.
8. Aspirate until negative pressure is reached. If negative pressure is never obtained, a tension pneumothorax may be present, and chest tubes with continuous suction are needed.

L-Thyroxine *see* Levothyroxine

NOTES

Tibial compression test [5]

Indications/Use

- To diagnose partial or complete rupture of the cranial cruciate ligament (CCL).
- NB Not all dogs with CCL disease have femorotibial instability that can be detected by this test.
- Often used in association with the cranial draw test.

Patient preparation and positioning

- Can be performed in the conscious animal. However, if the patient is tense (due to pain or temperament) or if the CCL is only partially torn, sedation or general anaesthesia is required.
- A conscious patient should be restrained in a standing position on three legs, with the affected limb held off the ground.
- Sedated or anaesthetized patients may be positioned in lateral recumbency, with the affected limb uppermost.

Technique

- Grasp and maintain the distal femur in a fixed position with one hand, placing the thumb over the lateral fabella and the index finger lightly on the tibial crest.
- Use the other hand to grasp the metatarsal region.
- Maintain the stifle joint in slight flexion, while slowly flexing the hock.

Tibia thrust

Results

- Cranial displacement (tibial thrust) of the tibial crest relative to the femur is suggestive of CCL injury.

See also Cranial draw test

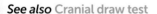

Tracheostomy [12]

1. The patient should be anaesthetized and an endotracheal tube placed. Depending on the nature of the upper airway disease, the size of the endotracheal tube may be significantly smaller than is expected for the size of the patient.
2. Place the patient in dorsal recumbency, with the neck extended. A sand bag placed beneath the neck will help with positioning. The ventral cervical region should be clipped and aseptically prepared if time permits.
3. A ventral cervical midline incision is made from the caudal aspect of the cricoid cartilage to the sixth tracheal ring.
4. The sternohyoid muscles are separated on the midline and retracted laterally.
5. The trachea should be isolated and a full-thickness stab incision should be made through the annular ligament between the third and fourth tracheal rings.
6. The incision in the trachea is extended laterally so that approximately 50–60% of the tracheal circumference is incised.
7. A tracheostomy tube approximately 50% of the tracheal diameter is placed into the lumen. The endotracheal tube must be withdrawn immediately prior to tracheostomy tube insertion.
8. Two stay sutures are placed in the rings adjacent to the tracheostomy site to facilitate exposure for placement of the tracheostomy tube.
9. The subcutaneous tissues and skin are apposed cranial and caudal to the tracheostomy site allowing a large enough opening for re-intubation if necessary. The tube is then secured with umbilical tape tied around the neck.
   - Patients with a temporary tracheostomy require careful 24-hour monitoring due to the risk of tube occlusion or dislodgement. Sterile technique should be used when handling the site, tracheostomy tubes and suction catheters.

⥤

- Postoperative care includes nebulization of the tube site to humidify the airways, frequent removal and cleaning of the inner cannula (if present) to prevent obstruction with mucus, and observation for swelling and irritation. Regular suctioning of the airway is no longer recommended.
- Short-term complications can include haemorrhage, obstruction of the tube, dislodgement, infection and damage to the peritracheal structures.

NOTES

Tramadol [25, 26]

(Tramadol ER*, Ultracet*, Ultram*, Zamadol*) POM CD Schedule 3

Formulations:

- Oral: 50 mg tablets; 100 mg, 200 mg, 300 mg immediate release tablets; sustained release tablets are also available in various tablet sizes; smaller tablet sizes (10 mg, 25 mg) are available from some veterinary wholesalers; 5 mg/ml oral liquid.
- Injectable: 50 mg/ml solution (may be difficult to source in the UK).

DOSES

Dogs: 2–5 mg/kg p.o. q8h, 2 mg/kg i.v.

Cats: 2–4 mg/kg p.o. q8h, 1–2 mg/kg i.v., s.c.

Mammals:

- Primates: 2 mg/kg p.o., s.c., i.v. q12h
- Ferrets 5 mg/kg p.o., s.c. q12–24h
- Rabbits: 3–10 mg/kg p.o. q8–12h (note: analgesic dose not determined)
- Rats: 10–20 mg/kg p.o., s.c. q8–12h
- Mice: 10–40 mg/kg s.c. q12h.

Birds:

- Bald eagles: 5 mg/kg p.o. q12h
- Hispaniolan Amazon parrots: 30 mg/kg p.o. q6h to achieve human therapeutic levels. Reduced thermal withdrawal response for 6 hours post-dosing
- Red-tailed hawks: 15 mg/kg p.o. q12h to achieve human therapeutic levels.

Reptiles:

- Red-eared sliders: 5–10 mg/kg i.m., p.o. q24–48h
- Bearded dragons: 11 mg/kg p.o.

Amphibians, Fish: No information available.

Tremors — differential diagnoses [15]

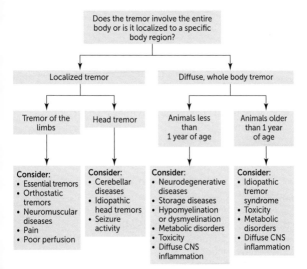

Does the tremor involve the entire body or is it localized to a specific body region?

Localized tremor

- **Tremor of the limbs**
  - **Consider:**
    - Essential tremors
    - Orthostatic tremors
    - Neuromuscular diseases
    - Pain
    - Poor perfusion

- **Head tremor**
  - **Consider:**
    - Cerebellar diseases
    - Idiopathic head tremors
    - Seizure activity

Diffuse, whole body tremor

- **Animals less than 1 year of age**
  - **Consider:**
    - Neurodegenerative diseases
    - Storage diseases
    - Hypomyelination or dysmyelination
    - Metabolic disorders
    - Toxicity
    - Diffuse CNS inflammation

- **Animals older than 1 year of age**
  - **Consider:**
    - Idiopathic tremor syndrome
    - Toxicity
    - Metabolic disorders
    - Diffuse CNS inflammation

Trilostane [25, 26]

(Vetoryl) POM-V

Formulations: Oral: 10 mg, 30 mg, 60 mg, 120 mg capsules. 5 mg capsules are available on a named patient basis.

DOSES

Dogs: Hyperadrenocorticism: 2 mg/kg p.o. q24h.

Cats: Hyperadrenocorticism: 30 mg/cat p.o. q24h.

Mammals: Rodents: 2–4 mg/kg p.o. q24h.

Birds, Reptiles, Amphibians, Fish: No information available.

NOTES

Urethral catheterization – male cat [12]

- Sedation is generally required unless the patient is paralysed or moribund.
- Place the cat in lateral recumbency.
- Clip and aseptically prepare the perineal area.
- Aseptically prepare hands and wear sterile gloves.
- A silicone-coated urinary catheter is less irritant than polypropylene. Open-ended catheters (rather than those with side openings) allow easier flushing. Sterile lubricant should be placed on the end of the catheter.
- Retract the prepuce and hold in place cranially between the forefinger and thumb of the non-dominant hand (this can be performed by an assistant).
- Place the tip of the urinary catheter into the urethra and gently advance approximately 0.5 cm. If you are unable to place the catheter into the tip of the urethra, gently massage the tip of the penis; occasionally there is a mucoid plug right at the tip which prevents placement.
- If any resistance is noted then flush the catheter with sterile saline.
- Once the catheter is in the urethra, allow the prepuce to return to its resting position and then gently pull the prepuce caudally. This allows alignment of the penile and membranous urethrae and thereby eases passage of the catheter.
- Advance the catheter gently, flushing with sterile saline if any resistance is encountered. Gentle rotation of the catheter may aid advancement.
- Once the catheter is in the bladder, suture the catheter to the perineal region. Drain urine from the bladder using a syringe, taking any samples required.
- If the cat was suffering from urethral obstruction then flush the bladder with warmed sterile saline until the fluid draining is no longer sanguineous.
- Attach a collection bag (a dry, clean, empty fluid bag and giving set is acceptable if a purpose-designed bag is not available) to the urinary catheter and

tape the catheter to the cat's tail to decrease any drag on the perineum and penis.
- Place the collection bag on a clean incontinence pad on the floor or hook to a kennel door lower than the patient to allow free urine drainage.
- Alternatively, bung the urinary catheter.
- DO NOT leave the urinary catheter open.
- Drain urine in a sterile fashion every 4 hours and record the volume produced.
- Place an Elizabethan collar on the cat.

NOTES

Urinalysis – dog and cat [9]

Parameter	Normal value	Abnormal value
pH	6.0–7.5	>7.5 <6.0
Glucose	Negative	Trace or positive
Ketones	Negative	1+ or greater
Bilirubin	Dogs: negative, trace or 1+, depending on urine concentration Cats: negative	Dogs: 2+ or above Cats: trace or above
Blood	Negative	Positive
Haemoglobin	Negative	Positive
Protein	Negative or trace	1+ or greater if urine dilute 2+ or greater if urine concentrated

Interpretation of urine dipstick results in dogs and cats.

Sediment constituent	Expected quantity (from centrifugation of 5 ml urine)	Comments
Leucocytes	<5 per hpf (X400)	Some microscopes may not have a standard-sized field of view
Erythrocytes	<5 per hpf (X400)	
Epithelial cells	0–2 per lpf (X100)	Small cells from kidney and upper tract; large cells from bladder and urethra
Bacteria	None	>1 x 10^4/ml rods or >1 x 10^5/ml cocci must be present to enable detection on sediment examination
Casts	Usually none	Low numbers of hyaline casts or rare granular casts can be seen in healthy animals
Crystals		Many types of crystal can be found in normal animals; their presence does not necessarily indicate a pathological state

Expected sediment findings in urine from healthy dogs and cats.
hpf = high power field; lpf = low power field.

Urinalysis – rabbit [24]

Parameter	Normal findings	Comments
Urine volume	130 ml/kg per day	Urination usually sporadic in large volumes
Specific gravity	1.003–1.036	Ability to concentrate urine is useful in assessing renal function
Average pH	8.2	Sample must be freshly tested as bacteria can alter pH; can drop to 6 in anorexic rabbits
Crystals	Ammonium magnesium phosphate; calcium carbonate; calcium oxalate	Presence of large amounts of crystals in rabbit urine is not indicative of urinary tract disease
Casts, epithelial cells or bacteria	Absent to rare	If negative for bacteria does not rule out an infection; *Staphylococcus*, *Klebsiella* and *Pseudomonas* most common isolates; casts are rare in rabbits due to dissolution in alkaline urine
Leucocytes or erythrocytes	Occasionally present	Leucocytes indicate inflammation of the urinary tract; erythrocytes indicate inflammation or haemorrhage of the urogenital tract
Albumin	Occasionally present (especially in young rabbits)	If elevated may indicate renal damage, particularly if urine is dilute; check protein:creatinine ratio (UPC) and sediment analysis; can be renal or post-renal in origin
Glucose	Trace may be present	Increased if stressed
Ketones	Negative	May be found in anorexic rabbits

Urine specific gravity [9]

Specific gravity (SG)	Interpretation
1.015–1.045 1.035–1.060	Normal for dogs Normal for cats
Isosthenuria: 1.008–1.012	This is the concentration of plasma, and implies the kidneys are not changing the SG. The SG can fall within this range with many conditions that cause PU/PD or in normal animals in certain circumstances. SG in this range with azotaemia supports a diagnosis of renal failure
Dilute urine (hyposthenuria): <1.008	This implies the kidneys can alter SG and make urine more dilute, and therefore excludes renal failure. Possible causes include diabetes insipidus, primary polydipsia or conditions that interfere with the action of ADH
Concentrated urine: >1.030 in dog >1.035 in cat	Suggests kidney disease is not present. Useful to confirm prerenal azotaemia. Approximately two-thirds of nephron function must be lost before abnormalities in renal concentrating ability occur, therefore clinically inapparent renal disease could be present with concentrated urine
Partially concentrated urine: 1.013–1.029 in dog 1.013–1.034 in cat	May be partial impairment of renal function or partial deficiency/lack of response to ADH. If the animal is clinically dehydrated this is considered inappropriately dilute
Inappropriately dilute: <1.030 in dog <1.035 in cat With clinical evidence of dehydration or azotaemia	This can be due to renal disease, or a partial deficiency or incomplete action of ADH. Concurrent pre-renal azotaemia and a condition that causes a deficiency/reduced action of ADH is also possible
Inappropriately concentrated urine: >1.007 in an over-hydrated patient	Suggests there is renal disease because the kidneys should produce dilute urine in this situation

ADH = antidiuretic hormone; PU/PD = polyuria and polydipsia. (Modified from www.iris-kidney.com)

Uveitis causes [12]

Dog

- Trauma
- Lens-induced (phacolytic, phacoclastic uveitis or lens luxation)
- Ulcerative keratitis
- Scleritis (deep necrotizing or non-necrotizing)
- Neoplastic and paraneoplastic disorders:
  - Primary or secondary neoplasia (e.g. lymphoma, melanoma, carcinoma)
  - Histiocytic proliferative disease
  - Granulomatous meningoencephalitis (GME)
  - Hyperviscosity syndrome
- Infection:
  - Bacterial (septicaemia of any cause, *Brucella canis, Leptospira* spp., *Borrelia burgdorferi, Bartonella vinsonii*)
  - Protozoal (*Toxoplasma gondii, Leishmania infantum, Neospora caninum, Trypanosoma evansi*)
  - Fungal (*Aspergillus fumigatus, Blastomyces dermatitidis, Candida albicans, Coccidioides immitis, Cryptococcus neoformans, Histoplasmacapsulatum*)
  - Rickettsial diseases (*Ehrlichia canis, Anaplasma platys, Rickettsia rickettsia*)
  - Viral (adenovirus infection (including postvaccinal 'blue-eye'), canine distemper virus, canine herpesvirus)
  - Parasitic (*Cuterebra* spp., *Dirofilaria immitis, Angiostrongylus vasorum, Toxocara canis, Balisascaris* spp., *Onchocerca lupi, Encephalitozoon cuniculi*)
  - Algal (*Prototheca* spp.)
- Metabolic (e.g. systemic hypertension, coagulopathies, hyperlipidaemia)
- Immune-mediated disease (e.g. uveodermatological syndrome, immune-mediated thrombocytopenia, immune-mediated vasculitis)
- Pigmentary and cyst glaucoma in the Golden Retriever
- Toxaemia (e.g. pyometra)
- Drug-induced (particularly miotic and prostaglandin agents)
- Radiation therapy
- Idiopathic uveitis and exudative retinal detachment
- Idiopathic

Cat

- Trauma
- Primary or secondary neoplasia (e.g. lymphoma, diffuse iridal melanoma, sarcoma, carcinoma)
- Lens-induced (phacolytic, septic lens implantation syndrome or lens luxation)

Cat *continued*

- Ulcerative keratitis
- Infection:
  - Viral (feline leukaemia virus (FeLV), feline immunodeficiency virus (FIV), feline infectious peritonitis (FIP), feline herpesvirus-1).
  - Protozoal (*Toxoplasma gondii*, *Leishmania infantum*)
  - Bacterial (*septicaemia*, *Bartonella* spp.)
  - Fungal (*Blastomyces dermatitidis*, *Coccidioides immitis*, *Cryptococcus neoformans*, *Histoplasma capsulatum*)
  - Parasitic (*Cuterebra* spp., *Encephalitozoon cuniculi*)
- Metabolic (e.g. systemic hypertension, coagulopathies, hyperlipidaemia)
- Idiopathic (chronic lymphoplasmacytic)
- Periarteritis

NOTES

NOTES

Vertebral heart score **see** Heart – vertebral heart score

NOTES

Wounds – emergency care [12]

- Haemostasis.
- Cover wound with sterile dressing whilst preparing for lavage.
- Wear sterile gloves (and hat, mask, gown).
- Apply gel or sterile saline-soaked swabs to the wound.
- Clip away hair, working from wound outwards if possible.
- Flush wound with sterile saline, remove all contaminants from chemical burns.
- Take a bacterial swab for culture.
- Apply a sterile dressing and bandage.

NOTES

Wounds – recognition and treatment [12]

Wound type	Description	Treatment considerations
Abrasion	Superficial wound involving destruction of tissues of varying depths of skin by friction or shearing forces. Usually bleeds minimally	When associated with a fracture, normal skin barrier is incompetent – treat fracture as grade I open
Avulsion	Characterized by tearing of tissues from attachments and creation of skin flaps. Limb avulsion injuries with extensive skin loss are called 'degloving'	Blood supply to skin may be compromised, leading to skin necrosis 2–5 days after injury. Repeat examinations and consider secondary debridement
Bite wound	A wound received from the teeth of an animal. Can cause a combination of puncture wounds, penetrating trauma, tears and crushing of tissue	Serious haemorrhage can occur if major vessels are pierced. Infection can occur from the pathogens in the biter's mouth
Burn – chemical	Direct exposure to noxious chemicals	Copious lavage to remove chemical. Ensure animal cannot lick area and ingest harmful substances
Burn – thermal	May see reddened, crusted or blackened skin. Burn injuries around the head and neck may compromise respiration	Beware of systemic complications of the burn. Attend to analgesia and cooling the area
Contusion	Blunt trauma may cause blood to pool in the subcutaneous tissue	Application of cold and analgesics. Beware of compartment syndrome
Crushing injuries	Combination of other injuries with extensive damage and contusion to the skin and deeper tissues	Assess neurological and vascular supply prior to treatment

Gunshots	These are contaminated. The heat generated in firing a bullet does not render it sterile. Open fractures may be present	Remove metal if encountered but not usually necessary to remove all fragments unless intra-articular or impinging on major structures such as nerves and arteries. Antibiosis for severe or intra-articular injuries. Treat the wound not the weapon
Laceration	Created by tearing, which damages the skin and underlying tissues and may be superficial or deep and have irregular edges	Debridement and primary closure may be used if treatment is early
Penetrating foreign body	Foreign bodies such as sticks and glass can fragment, causing widespread contamination	May need extensive exploration to remove all fragments (90% of glass shards show on radiographs). Protruding foreign bodies should be left in place for transport but can be cut 2–3 cm from the body but to minimize further internal damage by preventing the protruding shaft acting as a fulcrum
Penetrating trauma (e.g. stabbing)	Penetrating trauma is an injury that occurs when an object pierces the skin and enters a tissue of the body, creating an open wound. There may be an entry and exit hole	If abdominal or thoracic wound, check vital signs as there may be significant haemorrhage. Penetrating abdominal wounds require exploratory laparotomy
Puncture wound	A puncture wound is caused by an object piercing the skin and creating a small hole, which can be closed over and be barely visible. There is no exit wound. Damage can be superficial or deep	Infection may occur as the small puncture in the skin rapidly seals over. To treat the injury, the hole may need to be enlarged and opened, and the wound may need exploration for a foreign body such as a splinter

NOTES

Xylitol poisoning (URGENT) [1]

Also known as: Food additive E967

Description/exposure

Xylitol is a natural, sugar-free sweetener commonly found in diabetic chewing gum, calorie-free products (e.g. chewing gum, snacks, sweets), chewable multivitamins, over-the-counter (OTC) or prescription supplements or medications, food products (e.g. baked goods, peanut butter) and common household products (e.g. nasal spray, mouthwash, toothpaste).

Mechanism of action

In non-primate species, xylitol results in an insulin spike within 15–30 minutes of ingestion which causes severe hypoglycaemia. In dogs, doses as low as 0.05–0.1 g/kg have been associated with hypoglycaemia. With higher doses (>0.5 g/kg), acute hepatic necrosis can be seen.

Clinical presentation

Patients typically present with clinical signs of hypoglycaemia, including lethargy, vomiting, weakness, collapse, tremors and seizures. In patients ingesting hepatotoxic doses, clinical signs of malaise, melena, icterus, gastrointestinal distress, lethargy, collapse, coagulopathy, altered mentation (secondary to hepatic encephalopathy) and seizures may be seen.

Diagnostics

On initial presentation, a blood glucose level should be measured. Frequent blood glucose monitoring is recommended. In patients ingesting a potentially hepatotoxic dose of xylitol, baseline haematology and biochemistry should be performed. If hepatotoxicity occurs, clinicopathological changes may include hyperbilirubinaemia, elevated liver enzymes, hypoglycaemia, hypoalbuminaemia, hypocholesterolaemia, decreased blood urea nitrogen (BUN), hyperammonaemia and prolonged clotting times. ⇢

Treatment

Hypoglycaemic patients should receive an immediate bolus of 50% glucose or dextrose (1 g/kg), diluted with an equal volume of 0.9% NaCl or lactated Ringer's solution (given intravenously over 1–2 minutes). Once the patient is stable and normoglycaemic, induction of emesis can be considered if a large wad of gum is suspected to have formed a bezoar in the stomach. Activated charcoal does not need to be administered to animals with xylitol toxicosis as it is does not bind reliably. In hypoglycaemic patients, additional supplementation with a constant rate infusion of dextrose (2.5–5% dextrose in isotonic crystalloid maintenance fluids) should be continued for 12–24 hours, until the blood glucose level stabilizes. Patients that have ingested a dose considered to be hepatotoxic (>0.5 g/kg) should be treated with hepatoprotectants (e.g. SAMe, NAC, milk thistle), supportive care and monitoring of liver enzyme concentrations.

Prognosis

With hospitalization and supportive care, the outcome is fair. Liver failure is less common due to pet owner awareness, but can be severe and potentially fatal.

NOTES

NOTES

NOTES

References

1. *BSAVA (2018) Poisons database*. Available at: https://www.bsava.com/MyBSAVA/Knowledge-bank/Practice/Poisons-database

2. *BSAVA* **Companion**: How to approach the hypertensive patient (March 2012), by R.E. Jepson

3. *BSAVA* **Companion**: How to Perform effective cardiopulmonary resuscitation (August 2010), by S. Tappin

4. *BSAVA* **Companion**: How to Place an oesophagostomy tube (2012), by N. Bexfield and P. Watson

5. *BSAVA Guide to Procedures in Small Animal Practice, 2nd edn* (2014), ed. N. Bexfield and K. Lee

6. *BSAVA Manual of Canine and Feline Abdominal Surgery, 2nd edn* (2015), ed. J.M. Williams and J.D. Niles

7. *BSAVA Manual of Canine and Feline Anaesthesia and Analgesia, 3rd edn* (2016), ed. T. Duke-Novakovski, M. de Vries and C. Seymour

8. *BSAVA Manual of Canine and Feline Cardiorespiratory Medicine, 2nd edn* (2010), ed. V.L. Fuentes, L.R. Johnson and S. Dennis

9. *BSAVA Manual of Canine and Feline Clinical Pathology, 3rd edn* (2016), ed. E. Villiers and J. Ristić

10. *BSAVA Manual of Canine and Feline Dentistry and Oral Surgery, 4th edn* (2018), ed. A.M. Reiter and M. Gracis

11. *BSAVA Manual of Canine and Feline Dermatology, 3rd edn* (2012), ed. H.A. Jackson and R. Marsella

12. *BSAVA Manual of Canine and Feline Emergency and Critical Care, 3rd edn* (2018), ed. L.G. King and A. Boag

13. *BSAVA Manual of Canine and Feline Musculoskeletal Disorders, 2nd edn* (2018), ed. G. Arthurs, G. Brown and R. Pettitt

14. *BSAVA Manual of Canine and Feline Nephrology and Urology, 3rd edn* (2017), ed. J. Elliott, G.F. Grauer and J.L. Westropp

15. *BSAVA Manual of Canine and Feline Neurology, 4th edn* (2013), ed. S.R. Platt and N.J. Olby

16. *BSAVA Manual of Canine and Feline Ophthalmology, 3rd edn* (2014), ed. D. Gould and G.J. McLellan

17. *BSAVA Manual of Canine and Feline Reproduction and Neonatology, 2nd edn* (2010), ed. G.C.W. England and A. von Heimendahl

18. *BSAVA Manual of Canine and Feline Surgical Principles* (2012), ed. S.J. Baines, V. Lipscomb and T. Hutchinson

19. *BSAVA Manual of Canine and Feline Thoracic Imaging* (2008), ed.
    T. Schwarz and V. Johnson

20. *BSAVA Manual of Canine Practice* (2015), ed. T. Hutchinson and
    K. Robinson

21. *BSAVA Manual of Exotic Pets, 5th edn* (2010), ed. A. Meredith and
    C. Johnson-Delaney

22. *BSAVA Manual of Feline Practice* (2013), ed. A. Harvey and
    S. Tasker

23. *BSAVA Manual of Rabbit Medicine* (2014), ed. A. Meredith and
    B. Lord

24. *BSAVA Manual of Rabbit Surgery, Dentistry and Imaging* (2013),
    ed. F. Harcourt-Brown and J. Chitty

25. *BSAVA Small Animal Formulary – Part A: Canine and Feline,
    9th edn* (2017), editor-in-chief, I. Ramsey

26. *BSAVA Small Animal Formulary – Part B: Exotic Pets, 9th edn*
    (2015), editor-in-chief, A. Meredith

27. *BSAVA/VPIS Guide to Common Canine and Feline Poisons* (2012)

28. *Veterinary Ophthalmology, 4th edn* (2007), ed. K.N. Gelatt.
    Lippincott, Williams and Wilkins, Philadelphia

29. WSAVA (2013) *Body Condition Score charts.*
    Available at: http://www.wsava.org/Education-1/Global-
    Nutrition-Committee-Resources

Index of trade names

- 4fleas see Imidacloprid
- Acclaim spray see Methoprene
- ACP see Acepromazine
- Actidose-Aqua* see Charcoal
- Actrapid* see Insulin
- Adrenaline* see Adrenaline
- Advantage see Imidacloprid
- Advantix see Imidacloprid
- Advocate see Imidacloprid, Moxidectin
- Alvegesic see Butorphanol
- Alzane see Atipamezole
- Amfipen see Ampicillin
- Amitriptyline* see Amitriptyline
- Amlodipine* see Amlodipine
- Amodip see Amlodipine
- Amoxibactin see Amoxicillin
- Amoxycare see Amoxicillin
- Amoxypen see Amoxicillin
- Ampicare see Ampicillin
- Anesketin see Ketamine
- Antepsin* see Sucralfate
- Antepsin suspension* see Sucralfate
- Antirobe see Clindamycin
- Antisedan see Atipamezole
- Apometic see Apomorphine
- Apoquel see Oclacitinib
- Aquatet [Pharmaq] see Oxytetracycline
- Aspirin BP* see Aspirin
- Atipam see Atipamezole
- Augmentin* see Co-amoxiclav

- Aurizon see Dexamethasone
- Baytril see Enrofloxacin
- Benefortin see Benazepril
- Betamox see Amoxicillin
- Bimoxyl see Amoxicillin
- Bisolvon see Bromhexine
- Bob Martin Double Action Dewormer see Imidacloprid
- Bob Martin Easy to Use Wormer see Fenbendazole
- Bravecto see Fluralaner
- Broadline see Fipronil, Methoprene, Praziquantel
- Bupaq see Buprenorphine
- Buprecare see Buprenorphine
- Buprenodale see Buprenorphine
- Buprevet see Buprenorphine

- Canidryl see Carprofen
- Caninsulin see Insulin
- Carafate* see Sucralfate
- Cardalis see Benazepril
- Cardisure see Pimobendan
- Carprodyl see Carprofen
- Carprox Vet see Carprofen
- Cazitel see Praziquantel, Pyrantel
- Cefaseptin see Cefalexin
- Cephacare see Cefalexin
- Cephorum see Cefalexin
- Ceporex see Cefalexin
- Cerenia see Maropitant

– Certifect *see* Fipronil, Methoprene
– Cestem *see* Praziquantel, Pyrantel
– Charcodote* *see* Charcoal
– Cimetidine* *see* Cimetidine
– Clamoxyl *see* Amoxicillin
– Clavabactin *see* Co-amoxiclav
– Clavaseptin *see* Co-amoxiclav
– Clavucill *see* Co-amoxiclav
– Clavudale *see* Co-amoxiclav
– Clear Double Action Spot-on Solution *see* Imidacloprid
– Clearspot *see* Imidacloprid
– Clinacin *see* Clindamycin
– Clindacyl *see* Clindamycin
– Clindaseptin *see* Clindamycin
– ClinOleic* *see* Lipid infusions
– Codeine* *see* Codeine
– Combimox *see* Co-amoxiclav
– Combisyn *see* Co-amoxiclav
– Comfortan *see* Methadone
– Comfortis *see* Spinosad
– Convenia *see* Cefovecin
– Cydectin *see* Moxidectin

– Dexadreson *see* Dexamethasone
– Dexafort *see* Dexamethasone
– Dexa-ject *see* Dexamethasone

– Dexamethasone* *see* Dexamethasone
– Dexdomitor *see* Dexmedetomidine
– Diazemuls* *see* Diazepam
– Diazepam Rectubes* *see* Diazepam
– Dimazon *see* Furosemide
– Dolagis *see* Carprofen
– Dolorex *see* Butorphanol
– Dolpac *see* Praziquantel, Pyrantel
– Domitor *see* Medetomidine
– Dorbene *see* Medetomidine
– Dormilan *see* Medetomidine
– Doxyseptin 300 *see* Doxycycline
– Droncit *see* Praziquantel, Pyrantel
– Droncit Spot-on *see* Praziquantel
– Drontal *see* Praziquantel, Pyrantel
– Duphacort *see* Dexamethasone
– Duphalac* *see* Lactulose
– Dyspamet* *see* Cimetidine

– Effipro *see* Fipronil
– Eliminall *see* Fipronil
– Emeprid *see* Metoclopramide
– EMLA *see* Lidocaine
– Endectrid *see* Moxidectin
– Endoguard *see* Praziquantel, Pyrantel
– Engemycin *see* Oxytetracycline
– Enrocare *see* Enrofloxacin

* Products that are not authorized for veterinary use by the Veterinary Medicines Directorate

- Enrotab *see* Enrofloxacin
- Enrotron *see* Enrofloxacin
- Enrox *see* Enrofloxacin
- Enroxil *see* Enrofloxacin
- Epinephrine* *see* Adrenaline

- Felevox *see* Fipronil
- Felimazole *see* Methimazole
- Fenoflox *see* Enrofloxacin
- Fiprospot *see* Fipronil
- Flagyl* *see* Metronidazole
- Floxabactin *see* Enrofloxacin
- Floxibac *see* Enrofloxacin
- Fluke-Solve *see* Praziquantel
- Fortekor *see* Benazepril
- Fortekor-Plus *see* Benazepril, Pimobendan
- Frontect *see* Fipronil
- Frontline Combo/Plus *see* Methoprene
- Frontline *see* Fipronil
- Frusecare *see* Furosemide
- Frusedale *see* Furosemide
- Frusol* *see* Furosemide

- Galastop *see* Cabergoline
- Gastrogard *see* Omeprazole
- Granofen *see* Fenbendazole

- Humulin* *see* Insulin
- Hypurin* *see* Insulin

- Inflacam *see* Meloxicam
- Insulatard* *see* Insulin
- Intralipid* *see* Lipid infusions
- Intubeaze *see* Lidocaine
- Istin* *see* Amlodipine
- Ivelip* *see* Lipid infusions

- Kaminox *see* Potassium salts
- Kelactin *see* Cabergoline
- Kelapril *see* Benazepril
- Kesium *see* Co-amoxiclav
- Ketaset injection *see* Ketamine
- Ketavet *see* Ketamine

- Lactugal* *see* Lactulose
- Lactulose* *see* Lactulose
- Laevolac* *see* Lactulose
- Lantus* *see* Insulin
- Lapizole *see* Fenbendazole
- Leventa *see* Levothyroxine
- Libeo *see* Furosemide
- Lidoderm *see* Lidocaine
- Lignadrin *see* Lidocaine
- Lignol *see* Lidocaine
- Lipidem* *see* Lipid infusions
- Lipofundin* *see* Lipid infusions
- Liqui-Char* *see* Charcoal
- Locaine *see* Lidocaine
- Locovetic *see* Lidocaine
- Losec* *see* Omeprazole
- Loxicom *see* Meloxicam

- Maxidex* *see* Dexamethasone
- Maxitrol* *see* Dexamethasone
- Maxolon* *see* Metoclopramide
- Medetor *see* Medetomidine
- Meloxidyl *see* Meloxicam
- Meloxivet *see* Meloxicam
- Mepradec* *see* Omeprazole
- Metacam *see* Meloxicam
- Metoclopramide* *see* Metoclopramide

⟱

- Metomotyl see Metoclopramide
- Metrobactin see Metronidazole
- Metrolyl* see Metronidazole
- Metronidazole* see Metronidazole
- Milbactor see Praziquantel
- Milbemax see Milbemycin, Praziquantel
- Milpro see Praziquantel
- Multi-parasite see Moxidectin
- Mycinor see Clindamycin

- Narketan-10 see Ketamine
- Nelio see Benazepril
- Neurontin* see Gabapentin
- Nexguard Spectra see Milbemycin
- Nisamox see Co-amoxiclav
- Nisinject see Co-amoxiclav
- Noroclav see Co-amoxiclav

- Omegaven* see Lipid infusions
- Onsior see Robenacoxib
- Ornicure see Doxycycline
- Otimectin Vet see Ivermectin
- Oxycare see Oxytetracycline
- Oxytocin S see Oxytocin

- Panacur see Fenbendazole
- Paracetamol see Paracetamol
- Pardale V see Paracetamol, Codeine

- Perfalgan see Paracetamol
- Pimocard see Pimobendan
- Piriton* see Chlorphenamine
- PLT see Prednisolone
- Powerflox see Enrofloxacin
- Prazitel see Praziquantel, Pyrantel
- Pred-forte* see Prednisolone
- Prednicare see Prednisolone
- Prednidale see Prednisolone
- Previcox see Firocoxib
- Prilben see Benazepril
- Prinovox see Moxidectin
- Profender see Praziquantel
- Program see Lufenuron
- Program plus see Lufenuron, Milbemycin
- Promeris see Metaflumizone
- Promeris Duo see Metaflumizone
- Prozinc see Insulin
- Pulmodox see Doxycycline

- Quinoflox see Enrofloxacin

- R.I.P. fleas see Methoprene
- Ranitidine* see Ranitidine
- Rapidexon see Dexamethasone
- Revertor see Atipamezole
- Revitacam see Meloxicam
- Rheumocam see Meloxicam
- Rilexine see Cefalexin
- Rimadyl see Carprofen
- Rimifin see Carprofen
- Ronaxan see Doxycycline

* Products that are not authorized for veterinary use by the Veterinary Medicines Directorate

- Sedastart see Medetomidine
- Sedastop see Atipamezole
- Sedator see Medetomidine
- Sededorm see Medetomidine
- Semintra see Telmisartan
- Sileo see Dexmedetomidine
- Soloxine see Levothyroxine
- Staykill see Methoprene
- Stesolid* see Diazepam
- Stomorgyl see Metronidazole
- Stronghold see Selamectin
- Synuclav see Co-amoxiclav
- Synulox see Co-amoxiclav

- Tagamet* see Cimetidine
- Tardak see Delmadinone
- Therios see Cefalexin
- Thyforon see Levothyroxine
- Thyronorm see Methimazole
- Tipafar see Atipamezole
- Torbugesic see Butorphanol
- Torbutrol see Butorphanol
- Torphasol see Butorphanol
- Tramadol ER* see Tramadol
- Trifexis see Milbemycin, Spinosad
- Tsefalen see Cefalexin
- Tumil-K see Potassium salts
- Twinox see Co-amoxiclav

- Ultracet* see Tramadol
- Ultram* see Tramadol

- Valium* see Diazepam
- Veloxa see Praziquantel, Pyrantel
- Vetalar-V see Ketamine
- Vetergesic see Buprenorphine
- Vetmedin see Pimobendan
- Vetoryl see Trilostane
- Vetpril see Benazepril
- Vibramycin* see Doxycycline
- Vibravenos* see Doxycycline
- Vidalta see Carbimazole
- Vomend see Metoclopramide
- Voren see Dexamethasone

- Xeden see Enrofloxacin

- Zamadol* see Tramadol
- Zanprol* see Omeprazole
- Zantac* see Ranitidine
- Zerofen see Fenbendazole
- Zitac see Cimetidine
- Zobuxa see Enrofloxacin

ALWAYS read the relevant monographs

Cardiac emergencies

- **Asystole or pulseless electrical activity**
  - Adrenaline: 10 µg (micrograms)/kg i.v every 3–5 minutes until return of spontaneous circulation – this is equivalent to 1 ml/10 kg using 1:10,000 concentration (100 µg/ml). Double dose if used intratracheally.
- **Hyperkalaemic myocardial toxicity**
  - Calcium: 50–150 mg/kg calcium (boro)gluconate = 0.5–1.5 ml/kg of a 10% solution i.v. over 20–30 min *or* Soluble insulin: 0.5 IU/kg i.v. followed by 2–3 g of dextrose/unit of insulin (for urinary tract obstruction but not hypoadrenocorticism). Half the dextrose should be given as a bolus and the remainder administered i.v. over 4–6h.
- **Other bradyarrhythmias**
  - Atropine: 0.01–0.03 mg/kg i.v.– this is equivalent to 0.3–1 ml/20 kg using 0.6 mg/ml solution.
- **Ventricular tachycardia**
  - Lidocaine:
    Dogs: 2–8 mg/kg i.v. in 2 mg/kg boluses, followed by a constant rate i.v. infusion of 0.025–0.1 mg/kg/min.
    Cats: 0.25–2.0 mg/kg i.v. slowly in 0.25–0.5 mg/kg boluses followed by a constant rate i.v. infusion of 0.01–0.04 mg/kg/min.

Pulmonary emergencies

- **Respiratory arrest**
  - Doxapram: 5–10 mg/kg i.v., repeat according to need; duration of effect is approximately 15–20 min. Neonates: 1–2 drops under the tongue (oral solution) or 0.1 ml i.v. into the umbilical vein; this should be used only once.